The *Dr. Now*

1200-CALORIE DIET PLAN

A Proven Path to Weight Loss and Better Health with Dr. Nowzaradan's Balanced Meal Formula—365 Days of Easy, Affordable, and Delicious Recipes

Ella Claire Reed

TABLE OF CONTENTS

INTRODUCTION

Obesity is a modern-day epidemic affecting millions of people worldwide. The journey to a healthier life is often filled with countless obstacles, misinformation, and emotional struggles. My own path as a dietitian and writer has been deeply influenced by the stories of resilience and transformation I've witnessed over the years. One figure who has consistently stood out in the battle against obesity is Dr. Younan Nowzaradan, affectionately known as Dr. Now. His groundbreaking work in bariatric surgery and his compassionate approach to patient care have inspired countless individuals to reclaim their health and lives.

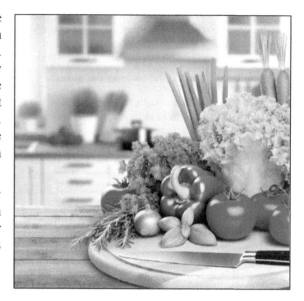

This book aims to provide a comprehensive guide to Dr. Now's dietary principles, offering practical advice and delicious recipes that align with his philosophy. Whether you are on the brink of starting your weight loss journey or seeking new ways to maintain your health, this book is designed to be a valuable resource.

Objectives of the Book

The primary goal of this book is to demystify the principles behind Dr. Now's approach to weight loss and health. We aim to achieve this through:

1. **Education**: Providing clear, evidence-based explanations of the fundamental principles of a healthy diet as advocated by Dr. Nowzaradan. Understanding the "why" behind dietary recommendations can make it easier to follow through and see results.
2. **Practical Guidance**: Offering step-by-step strategies for meal planning, portion control, and making healthier food choices. This includes tips on how to navigate common challenges and avoid pitfalls.
3. **Inspiration**: Sharing success stories of individuals who have transformed their lives through Dr. Now's guidance. These testimonials serve as powerful reminders that change is possible and can be sustained.
4. **Recipes**: Presenting a collection of nutritious, delicious, and easy-to-prepare recipes that adhere to Dr. Now's dietary guidelines. These recipes are designed to support weight loss and long-term health while being enjoyable to eat.
5. **Support**: Highlighting the importance of psychological and social support in the weight loss journey. We discuss strategies for staying motivated, dealing with setbacks, and building a supportive environment.

By the end of this book, you should have a solid understanding of the dietary principles that can help you lose weight and improve your health, as well as a collection of practical tools and recipes to help you implement these principles in your daily life.

WHO IS DR. YOUNAN NOWZARADAN?

Biography and Career

Dr. Younan Nowzaradan, often referred to as Dr. Now, is a renowned bariatric surgeon based in Houston, Texas. Born in Iran in 1944, Dr. Nowzaradan moved to the United States after completing his medical degree at the University of Tehran in 1970. He pursued further training in surgery and completed his residency at St. John Hospital in Detroit, Michigan. Dr. Nowzaradan is also a fellow of the American College of Surgeons.

Over the course of his career, Dr. Now has become a leading expert in the field of bariatric surgery, specializing in the treatment of morbid obesity. He is widely recognized for his work on the reality television show "My 600-lb Life," where he has helped countless individuals achieve life-changing weight loss through surgical intervention and rigorous dietary regimens. His compassionate yet straightforward approach has garnered him a dedicated following and has made him a respected figure in both the medical community and among the general public.

Contributions to Bariatric Surgery

Dr. Nowzaradan's contributions to bariatric surgery are significant and multifaceted. He has performed thousands of weight loss surgeries, including gastric bypass, sleeve gastrectomy, and laparoscopic procedures, often on patients deemed too high-risk by other surgeons. His willingness to take on these challenging cases has saved many lives and has pushed the boundaries of what is considered possible in bariatric surgery.

One of Dr. Now's key contributions is his development of a comprehensive pre- and post-operative care program. This program emphasizes the importance of diet and lifestyle changes in addition to surgical intervention. Dr. Now insists that surgery is not a magic bullet but a tool that must be used in conjunction with a strict dietary regimen and behavioral modifications to achieve lasting success. His approach has set a new standard in the field and has highlighted the critical role of multidisciplinary care in the treatment of obesity.

Dr. Now has also been a vocal advocate for the destigmatization of obesity. He consistently emphasizes that obesity is a complex, chronic disease influenced by genetic, environmental, and psychological factors. By treating his patients with respect and compassion, he challenges the biases and prejudices that many obese individuals face. His work has helped to shift public perception and has encouraged more empathetic and comprehensive approaches to obesity treatment.

Dr. Now's Philosophy

At the heart of Dr. Nowzaradan's philosophy is the belief that everyone deserves a chance to improve their health and quality of life, regardless of their current weight or medical condition. His approach is grounded in several core principles:

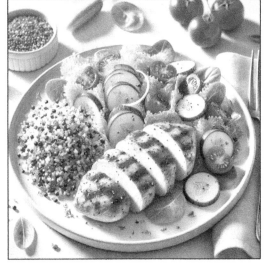

1. **Honesty and Accountability**: Dr. Now believes that honesty is crucial for successful weight loss. This means being truthful with oneself about eating habits and being accountable for one's actions. He often tells his patients that the scale does not lie, and that facing the reality of their situation is the first step toward change.
2. **Comprehensive Care**: Dr. Now's approach integrates medical, nutritional, and psychological support. He understands that obesity is a multifaceted disease that requires a holistic treatment plan. His patients receive not only surgical intervention but also dietary counseling, psychological support, and regular follow-ups to monitor their progress.
3. **Patient Empowerment**: Dr. Now empowers his patients by providing them with the knowledge and tools they need to take control of their health. He educates them about the science of nutrition, the importance of portion control, and the benefits of physical activity. By giving his patients the information they need, he helps them to make informed decisions and to develop sustainable healthy habits.
4. **Realistic Goals**: Dr. Now sets realistic and achievable goals for his patients. He recognizes that weight loss is a gradual process and encourages his patients to focus on steady, consistent progress rather than quick fixes. This strategy guarantees long-term success and fosters confidence.
5. **Compassion and Support**: Dr. Now's compassion for his patients is evident in his work. He provides unwavering support and encouragement, even in the face of setbacks and challenges. His patients often describe him as a source of hope and inspiration, and his dedication to their well-being is a testament to his commitment as a physician.

THE IMPORTANCE OF A HEALTHY DIET

Why a Balanced Diet is Crucial for Health

A balanced diet is the cornerstone of good health and well-being. It provides the body with the essential nutrients it needs to function correctly, maintain energy levels, and promote growth and repair. A balanced diet includes a variety of foods in the right proportions: carbohydrates, proteins, fats, vitamins, and minerals. Each of these components plays a vital role in supporting the body's complex systems and processes.

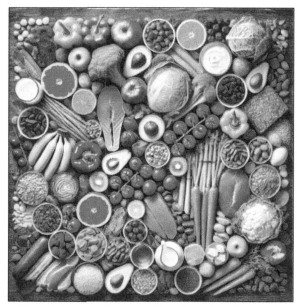

The body uses carbohydrates as its main energy source to power everything from routine tasks to strenuous exercise. Proteins are essential for building and repairing tissues, making enzymes, hormones, and other body chemicals. Fats, though often misunderstood, are crucial for brain health, energy, and the absorption of certain vitamins. Vitamins and minerals support a wide range of physiological functions, including immune response, bone health, and fluid balance.

When the diet is balanced, the body can function optimally, warding off disease, maintaining a healthy weight, and promoting overall well-being. Conversely, an imbalanced diet can lead to a host of health issues, from nutrient deficiencies to chronic diseases. Understanding and adopting the principles of a balanced diet is a fundamental step toward achieving and maintaining good health.

Impacts of Obesity on Physical and Mental Health

Obesity is a condition characterized by excessive body fat accumulation, which can have severe repercussions on both physical and mental health. Physically, obesity is linked to numerous chronic diseases and health conditions. It is a significant risk factor for type 2 diabetes, heart disease, stroke, and certain types of cancer. Obesity can also lead to hypertension (high blood pressure), dyslipidemia (high cholesterol levels), and sleep apnea.

The impact of obesity extends beyond these immediate health concerns. Excess body weight puts additional strain on the musculoskeletal system, leading to joint pain and osteoarthritis. It can impair respiratory function, making everyday activities more challenging and increasing the risk of respiratory illnesses. Moreover, obesity can weaken the immune system, making the body more susceptible to infections.

Mental health is equally affected by obesity. People who struggle with obesity frequently experience prejudice and stigma, which can result in low self-esteem and feelings of guilt and shame. These negative emotions can contribute to mental health disorders such as depression and anxiety. Additionally, the psychological stress of managing obesity can create a vicious cycle, where emotional eating exacerbates weight gain, further impacting mental health.

Children and adolescents with obesity are particularly vulnerable to these effects. They may experience bullying and social isolation, which can affect their academic performance and social development. The psychological impact of obesity in youth can persist into adulthood, highlighting the importance of early intervention and support.

Scientific Studies Supporting a Balanced Diet

The scientific community has extensively researched the benefits of a balanced diet, and the evidence is overwhelmingly positive. Numerous studies have demonstrated that a diet rich in fruits, vegetables, whole grains, lean proteins, and healthy fats can reduce the risk of chronic diseases and improve overall health.

A landmark study published in the New England Journal of Medicine found that adherence to a Mediterranean diet, characterized by high consumption of fruits, vegetables, nuts, and olive oil, significantly reduced the risk of cardiovascular events, such as heart attacks and strokes. The significance of including plant-based foods and healthy fats in the diet is highlighted by this study.

Research published in The Lancet highlights the global health benefits of a diet low in processed foods and high in whole, nutrient-dense foods. The study found that poor dietary habits are a leading cause of death and disability worldwide, surpassing even smoking. This reinforces the critical need for dietary interventions to improve public health outcomes.

The Dietary Approaches to Stop Hypertension (DASH) diet, endorsed by the National Heart, Lung, and Blood Institute, has shown significant results in lowering blood pressure. In addition to modest portions of whole grains, fish, poultry, and nuts, the DASH diet places a strong emphasis on fruits, vegetables, and low-fat dairy products. This diet has been proven effective in managing hypertension and promoting cardiovascular health.

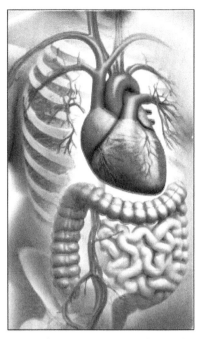

Furthermore, studies on dietary patterns have revealed that diets high in processed foods, sugars, and unhealthy fats are linked to increased risks of obesity, diabetes, and metabolic syndrome. In contrast, diets rich in fiber, antioxidants, and anti-inflammatory foods help in maintaining a healthy weight and reducing the risk of these chronic conditions.

In summary, the importance of a balanced diet is well-supported by scientific evidence. A diet that includes a variety of nutrient-dense foods can promote physical health, prevent chronic diseases, and support mental well-being.

FUNDAMENTAL PRINCIPLES OF DR. NOW'S DIET

Calories and Portion Control

One of the cornerstones of Dr. Nowzaradan's dietary philosophy is the meticulous control of calories and portion sizes. Understanding the relationship between calorie intake and weight management is crucial for anyone seeking to lose weight and maintain a healthy lifestyle. Dr. Now emphasizes that the number of calories consumed must be balanced with the number of calories burned through daily activities and exercise.

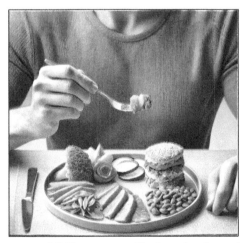

Portion control is a practical way to manage calorie intake without the need for extensive calorie counting, which can often be daunting and unsustainable for many individuals. Dr. Now advises using smaller plates and bowls to naturally reduce portion sizes. This simple yet effective strategy can help prevent overeating and encourages mindful eating practices. By being conscious of portion sizes, individuals can enjoy a variety of foods without exceeding their daily calorie limits.

Another key aspect of portion control is learning to listen to your body's hunger and fullness cues. Eating slowly and savoring each bite allows time for the body to signal when it is satisfied, reducing the likelihood of overeating. Dr. Now also recommends planning meals and snacks ahead of time to avoid impulsive eating and to ensure that portion sizes remain consistent.

Importance of Protein

Protein plays a vital role in Dr. Now's diet plan. It is a necessary macronutrient that promotes the synthesis of enzymes and hormones, immune system function, and muscle growth and repair. For individuals on a weight loss journey, protein is particularly beneficial because it helps to maintain muscle mass while losing fat, promotes satiety, and can boost metabolism.

Dr. Now recommends incorporating lean sources of protein into every meal. This includes options such as poultry, fish, eggs, low-fat dairy products, legumes, and tofu. These foods provide high-quality protein without the excess saturated fat found in some other protein sources. A typical meal might include a portion of grilled chicken breast, a serving of steamed vegetables, and a small side of quinoa, all of which contribute to a balanced intake of protein, fiber, and other nutrients.

In addition to whole foods, protein supplements such as shakes and bars can be useful, especially for those who have undergone bariatric surgery and may struggle to meet their protein needs through food alone. However, it is important to choose supplements that are low in added sugars and artificial ingredients.

Reducing Refined Carbohydrates and Sugars

Reducing the intake of refined carbohydrates and sugars is another fundamental principle of Dr. Now's diet. Refined carbohydrates, such as white bread, pastries, and sugary cereals, have been stripped of their nutritional value and can cause rapid spikes in blood sugar levels. These spikes are often followed by crashes that can lead to increased hunger and overeating.

Dr. Now advocates for a diet rich in whole, unprocessed foods. Whole grains like brown rice, quinoa, and oats are excellent alternatives to refined grains. These foods are higher in fiber, which slows down digestion and helps maintain steady blood sugar levels. Fiber also promotes a feeling of fullness, making it easier to stick to a calorie-controlled diet.

Sugars, particularly added sugars, should be minimized as much as possible. This means cutting back on sugary drinks, sweets, and processed foods that often contain hidden sugars. Reading food labels is crucial to identifying and avoiding products with high sugar content. Dr. Now suggests satisfying sweet cravings with natural sources of sweetness like fresh fruits, which also provide vitamins, minerals, and fiber.

Choosing Healthy Fats

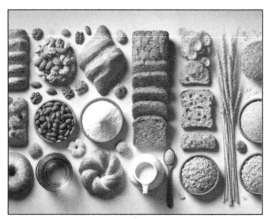

A balanced diet must include fats, but not all fats are created equal. Dr. Now emphasizes the importance of choosing healthy fats, which can support heart health, improve cholesterol levels, and provide long-lasting energy. Monounsaturated and polyunsaturated fats, which are present in foods like avocados, almonds, seeds, olive oil, and fatty fish like salmon and mackerel, are examples of healthy fats.

These fats are beneficial because they can help reduce inflammation and are associated with a lower risk of chronic diseases. For example, omega-3 fatty acids, a type of polyunsaturated fat found in fish, flaxseeds, and walnuts, have been shown to support brain health and reduce the risk of heart disease.

Conversely, Dr. Now advises limiting saturated and trans fats, which are commonly found in fried foods, baked goods, and processed snacks. These unhealthy fats can raise bad cholesterol levels and increase the risk of heart disease and other health problems. By focusing on healthy fat sources and minimizing unhealthy ones, individuals can support their overall health and weight loss goals.

The Importance of Hydration

Hydration is a critical yet often overlooked component of a healthy diet. Water is essential for nearly every function in the body, including digestion, nutrient absorption, and temperature regulation. Staying well-hydrated can also aid in weight loss by helping to control hunger and maintain metabolic processes.

Dr. Now recommends drinking plenty of water throughout the day, with a general guideline of at least eight 8-ounce glasses daily, although individual needs may vary based on factors such as activity level, climate, and overall health. Starting the day with a glass of water and carrying a reusable water bottle can help ensure consistent hydration.

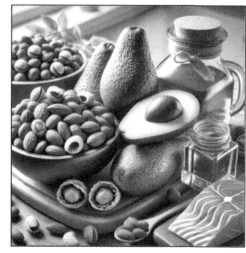

In addition to water, other hydrating beverages include herbal teas and water infused with fruits or vegetables like lemon, cucumber, and mint. It's important to limit the intake of sugary drinks, caffeinated beverages, and alcohol, which can lead to dehydration and add unnecessary calories to the diet.

For those who find it challenging to drink enough water, setting reminders or tracking intake through a mobile app can be helpful. Hydration not only supports physical health but also aids in maintaining mental clarity and energy levels, making it a vital aspect of Dr. Now's dietary approach.

STRUCTURING DR. NOW'S DIET

Creating a sustainable and effective diet plan can be a daunting task, but with the right approach and tools, it becomes a manageable and rewarding journey. Dr. Younan Nowzaradan's diet is designed to promote weight loss and improve overall health by focusing on balanced nutrition, portion control, and consistency. Here, we will explore the essential elements of structuring Dr. Now's diet, including meal planning, monitoring calorie intake, determining the frequency of meals and snacks, and making necessary adaptations for specific dietary needs.

Meal Planning

Meal planning is the cornerstone of any successful diet. It helps to ensure that you are consuming a balanced diet, staying within your calorie limits, and avoiding the temptation of unhealthy food choices. Dr. Now emphasizes the importance of planning meals ahead of time to maintain control over what you eat and to make healthier choices more convenient.

1. **Set Clear Goals**: Begin by setting clear, achievable goals. Whether it's losing a specific amount of weight, managing a health condition, or simply improving overall nutrition, having a goal will guide your meal planning process.
2. **Balanced Meals**: Ensure that each meal includes a balance of macronutrients: proteins, carbohydrates, and fats. Proteins should come from lean sources such as poultry, fish, legumes, and low-fat dairy. Carbohydrates should primarily be from whole grains, vegetables, and fruits, while fats should be healthy ones like those from avocados, nuts, seeds, and olive oil.
3. **Portion Control**: Portion control is critical in Dr. Now's diet. Use measuring cups, food scales, and portion guides to ensure you are consuming the right amounts of each food group. This helps prevent overeating and ensures you stay within your calorie limits.
4. **Variety**: Incorporate a variety of foods to ensure you get all the necessary nutrients. Different foods provide different vitamins and minerals, so a varied diet helps to cover all nutritional bases.
5. **Prep Ahead**: Prepare meals ahead of time to avoid last-minute unhealthy choices. Spend a few hours each week cooking and portioning meals so that healthy options are always available.

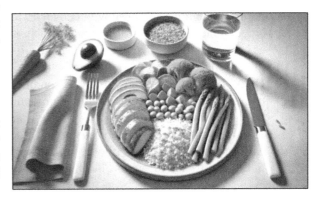

Monitoring Calorie Intake

Monitoring your calorie intake is essential to ensure you are not consuming more than your body needs. Dr. Now's diet typically recommends a low-calorie intake to facilitate weight loss, often around 1200 calories per day, depending on individual needs and medical conditions.

1. **Calculate Your Caloric Needs**: Use a calorie calculator to determine your daily caloric needs based on your age, gender, weight, height, and activity level. This will give you a baseline for how many calories you should consume to maintain your weight, and how much you need to reduce to lose weight.
2. **Track Your Intake**: Keep a food diary or use a calorie-tracking app to log everything you eat and drink. This helps you stay accountable and provides a clear picture of your eating habits.
3. **Read Labels**: Pay attention to food labels to understand the calorie content and nutritional value of packaged foods. Keep an eye out for added sodium, bad fats, and hidden sweets.
4. **Mindful Eating**: Practice mindful eating by paying attention to hunger and fullness cues, eating slowly, and savoring each bite. This can help prevent overeating and make you more aware of the quality and quantity of food you are consuming.

5. **Adjust as Needed**: Review your progress and calorie intake on a regular basis. If you are not losing weight as expected, you may need to adjust your calorie intake or increase your physical activity.

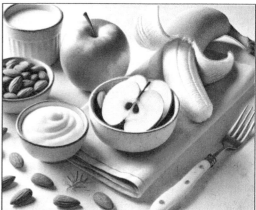

Frequency of Meals and Snacks

Dr. Nowzaradan advocates for regular meals and snacks to keep metabolism steady and prevent extreme hunger that can lead to overeating. The key is to find a meal frequency that works for you and helps you stay satisfied throughout the day.

1. **Three Main Meals**: Start with three balanced main meals—breakfast, lunch, and dinner. Each meal should include a good mix of protein, carbohydrates, and healthy fats to keep you full and energized.
2. **Healthy Snacks**: Include one or two healthy snacks between meals if needed. Snacks can help maintain energy levels and prevent overeating at the next meal. Choose snacks that are nutrient-dense and low in calories, such as a piece of fruit, a handful of nuts, or a serving of yogurt.
3. **Regular Intervals**: Try to eat at regular intervals, roughly every 3-4 hours. This helps to maintain blood sugar levels and prevents the extreme hunger that can lead to poor food choices.
4. **Listen to Your Body**: Be aware of the cues your body sends out regarding hunger and fullness. Eat when you are hungry and stop when you are content, not overly full. This helps to establish a healthy relationship with food and prevents the habit of eating out of boredom or stress.

Adaptations for Specific Dietary Needs

Every individual has unique dietary needs, whether due to medical conditions, allergies, or personal preferences. Dr. Now's diet can be adapted to accommodate these specific needs while still promoting weight loss and overall health.

1. **Diabetes**: For individuals with diabetes, it is important to manage blood sugar levels through diet. Focus on low-glycemic index foods that do not spike blood sugar levels. Include plenty of fiber-rich vegetables, whole grains, and lean proteins, and limit refined sugars and carbohydrates.
2. **Food Intolerances and Allergies**: Identify and avoid foods that trigger intolerances or allergies. Substitute with appropriate alternatives, such as using almond milk instead of cow's milk for those with lactose intolerance, or gluten-free grains for those with celiac disease.
3. **Vegetarian or Vegan Diets**: Ensure adequate protein intake by incorporating plant-based protein sources such as beans, lentils, tofu, tempeh, and quinoa. Pay attention to nutrients that may be lacking in a vegetarian or vegan diet, such as vitamin B12, iron, and omega-3 fatty acids, and consider supplements if necessary.
4. **Heart Health**: For those with heart conditions, focus on foods that support cardiovascular health. This includes plenty of fruits, vegetables, whole grains, and lean proteins. Limit saturated fats, trans fats, and sodium to reduce the risk of heart disease.
5. **Age-Related Nutritional Needs**: As we age, our nutritional needs change. Older adults may require more calcium and vitamin D for bone health, as well as more protein to maintain muscle mass. Ensure the diet is rich in these nutrients to support healthy aging.

KEY COMPONENTS OF DR. NOW'S DIET

In crafting a diet that promotes sustainable weight loss and overall health, Dr. Nowzaradan emphasizes the importance of balanced nutrition, portion control, and the quality of food choices. The key components of Dr. Now's diet include lean proteins, low-starch vegetables, whole grains, low-sugar fruits, and healthy fats. Each of these elements plays a crucial role in nourishing the body while supporting weight loss goals.

Lean Proteins: Poultry, Fish, Legumes

Lean proteins are the cornerstone of Dr. Now's dietary recommendations. Proteins are essential for building and repairing tissues, maintaining muscle mass, and supporting metabolic functions. By choosing lean sources of protein, you don't have to eat a lot of fat or calories to get the nutrients you need.

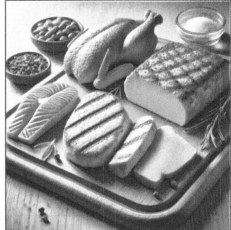

- **Poultry**: Lean protein can be found in abundance in chicken and turkey. They are versatile and can be prepared in a variety of healthy ways, such as grilling, baking, or broiling. Removing the skin and choosing white meat cuts, like the breast, helps reduce fat intake while maximizing protein content.
- **Fish**: Fish is not only a great source of lean protein but also rich in omega-3 fatty acids, which are beneficial for heart health. Dr. Now recommends incorporating fatty fish like salmon, mackerel, and sardines, as well as leaner options like cod and tilapia. For best results, try to have fish at least twice a week in your diet.
- **Legumes**: A great source of plant-based protein are beans, lentils, and peas. They are low in fat, high in fiber, and packed with essential nutrients. Legumes can be substituted for meat in a variety of recipes, including soups, stews, and salads. They provide a satisfying and nutritious alternative for vegetarians and those looking to reduce meat consumption.

Low-Starch Vegetables: Leafy Greens, Broccoli, Cauliflower

Vegetables are a critical component of any healthy diet, and Dr. Now places particular emphasis on low-starch varieties. These vegetables are low in calories and carbohydrates but high in vitamins, minerals, and fiber. They help keep you full and provide essential nutrients without adding extra calories.

- **Leafy Greens**: Spinach, kale, Swiss chard, and other leafy greens are nutrient-dense and incredibly low in calories. They can be incorporated into salads, smoothies, stir-fries, and soups. Leafy greens are high in antioxidants, which help protect your cells from damage and support overall health.
- **Broccoli**: Broccoli is a cruciferous vegetable known for its impressive nutritional profile. It is high in fiber, vitamins C and K, and contains compounds that have been shown to have cancer-fighting properties. Broccoli can be steamed, roasted, or added to various dishes for a nutritious boost.
- **Cauliflower**: Cauliflower is another versatile cruciferous vegetable that can be used as a low-carb substitute for grains and legumes. It can be riced, mashed, or roasted, providing a satisfying texture and flavor. Cauliflower is rich in vitamins C, K, and B6, and it supports digestive health with its high fiber content.

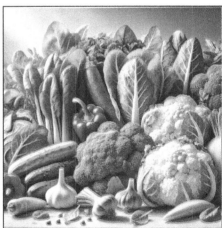

Whole Grains: Quinoa, Brown Rice, Oats

Whole grains are an essential part of Dr. Now's diet plan, providing sustained energy and important nutrients like fiber, vitamins, and minerals. Unlike refined grains, whole grains retain their bran and germ, offering more health benefits.

- **Quinoa**: Quinoa has all nine of the essential amino acids, making it a complete protein. It is also high in fiber, magnesium, and iron. Quinoa's versatility allows it to be used in salads, as a side dish, or as a base for bowls. Its nutty flavor and satisfying texture make it a popular choice for health-conscious individuals.
- **Brown Rice**: Because it is a whole grain, brown rice keeps its healthy bran and germ. It is a good source of magnesium, phosphorus, selenium, and B vitamins. Brown rice has a lower glycemic index compared to white rice, making it a better option for managing blood sugar levels. It goes well with soups and stir-fries among other foods.

- **Oats**: Oats are a fantastic whole grain option for breakfast or snacks. Because of their high soluble fiber content, they may help decrease cholesterol and promote heart health. Oats are also rich in vitamins and minerals, including manganese, phosphorus, and magnesium. Overnight oats, oatmeal, and oat-based smoothies are excellent ways to incorporate this grain into your diet.

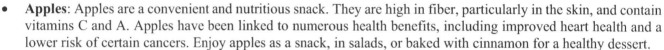

Low-Sugar Fruits: Berries, Apples, Citrus

Fruits provide essential vitamins, minerals, and antioxidants. Dr. Now advocates for low-sugar fruits to help manage calorie intake while still enjoying the sweet flavors and nutritional benefits fruits offer.

- **Berries**: Blackberries, raspberries, strawberries, and blueberries are rich in antioxidants and fiber but low in sugar. They are excellent for improving brain health, reducing inflammation, and providing essential vitamins like vitamin C and K. Berries can be added to cereals, yogurts, salads, or eaten on their own as a snack.
- **Apples**: Apples are a convenient and nutritious snack. They are high in fiber, particularly in the skin, and contain vitamins C and A. Apples have been linked to numerous health benefits, including improved heart health and a lower risk of certain cancers. Enjoy apples as a snack, in salads, or baked with cinnamon for a healthy dessert.
- **Citrus**: Citrus fruits like oranges, grapefruits, lemons, and limes are rich in vitamin C, fiber, and various antioxidants. They help with digestion, strengthen the immune system, and enhance skin health. Citrus fruits can be enjoyed on their own, added to salads, or used to flavor water and dishes.

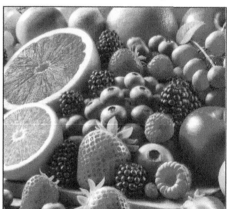

Healthy Fats: Avocado, Olive Oil, Nuts, and Seeds

Incorporating healthy fats into your diet is essential for overall health and satiety. Dr. Now emphasizes the importance of choosing sources of fats that provide health benefits rather than contributing to weight gain and health issues.

- **Avocado**: Avocado is a nutrient-dense fruit high in monounsaturated fats, which are heart-healthy. It also provides fiber, potassium, and vitamins C, E, and K. Avocado can be used in salads, sandwiches, smoothies, or as a spread on toast. Its creamy texture and rich flavor make it a satisfying addition to meals.
- **Olive Oil**: Olive oil is a staple of the Mediterranean diet, known for its numerous health benefits. It is high in monounsaturated fats and antioxidants, which can reduce inflammation and lower the risk of chronic diseases. Use olive oil for cooking, salad dressings, and as a finishing oil to add flavor to dishes.
- **Nuts and Seeds**: Almonds, walnuts, chia seeds, flaxseeds, and other nuts and seeds are excellent sources of healthy fats, protein, and fiber. They also contain important minerals and vitamins, including as omega-3 fatty acids, magnesium, and vitamin E. Nuts and seeds can be added to cereals, yogurts, salads, or enjoyed as a snack. Be mindful of portion sizes, as they are calorie-dense.

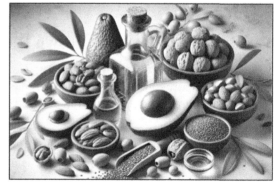

THE ROLE OF MEAL PREPARATION

Benefits of Meal Prep

Meal preparation, often abbreviated as "meal prep," is a cornerstone of effective weight management and healthy eating. By taking the time to plan and prepare meals in advance, you can gain control over your diet, reduce stress, and set yourself up for success. Here are some key benefits of meal prep:

1. **Consistency and Portion Control**: One of the biggest challenges in maintaining a healthy diet is ensuring consistent portion sizes. Meal prep allows you to portion out your meals ahead of time, ensuring that you are consuming the right amount of food without overeating. This is particularly important for weight loss and maintenance.
2. **Time and Stress Management**: Preparing meals in advance can save a significant amount of time during the week. Instead of scrambling to put together meals after a long day, you can simply reheat a pre-prepared dish. This reduces daily stress and frees up time for other important activities, such as exercise or relaxation.
3. **Nutritional Control**: When you prepare your own meals, you have complete control over the ingredients and cooking methods. This allows you to ensure that your meals are nutritious and aligned with your dietary goals. You can avoid hidden sugars, unhealthy fats, and excess sodium often found in processed and restaurant foods.
4. **Financial Savings**: Eating out or ordering takeout can be expensive. By prepping meals, you may cut down on food waste, take advantage of bargains, and purchase items in bulk. This can result in significant cost reductions over time.
5. **Improved Eating Habits**: Regular meal prep encourages healthier eating habits. By planning your meals, you are more likely to make thoughtful food choices rather than impulsive decisions based on convenience or cravings. This structured approach can help you stick to your dietary goals and avoid unhealthy snacks or meals.

Strategies for Efficient Preparation

Effective meal prep requires some planning and organization, but with the right strategies, it can become a seamless part of your routine. Here are some tips to help you get started:

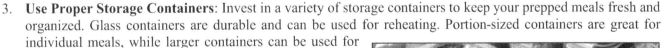

1. **Plan Your Meals**: Begin by planning your meals for the week. Consider your dietary goals, nutritional needs, and preferences. Aim for a balance of proteins, vegetables, whole grains, and healthy fats. Write down your meal plan and create a shopping list based on the ingredients you'll need.
2. **Batch Cooking**: Batch cooking involves preparing large quantities of food at once, which can then be divided into individual portions and stored for later use. This is a time-efficient way to ensure you have healthy meals ready to go. Examples of foods that can be batch cooked include grilled chicken, roasted vegetables, quinoa, and soups.
3. **Use Proper Storage Containers**: Invest in a variety of storage containers to keep your prepped meals fresh and organized. Glass containers are durable and can be used for reheating. Portion-sized containers are great for individual meals, while larger containers can be used for batch-cooked items.

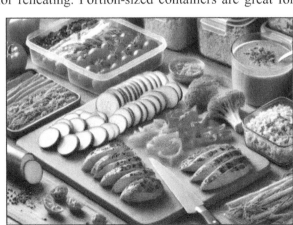

4. **Schedule Prep Time**: Set aside specific times during the week for meal prep. Many people find it helpful to prep on Sundays and Wednesdays, ensuring they have fresh meals for the entire week. Consider this time as a crucial appointment that you have with yourself.
5. **Prep Ingredients Separately**: If you prefer flexibility in your meals, consider prepping ingredients separately rather than assembling complete meals. For example, chop vegetables, cook proteins, and prepare grains. This allows you to mix and match ingredients to create different meals throughout the week.

6. **Simplify Recipes**: Choose simple recipes that are easy to prepare and don't require a lot of ingredients or complicated techniques. Focus on whole, minimally processed foods that can be prepared quickly.
7. **Label and Date Your Meals**: Label the contents and the preparation date on the label of each container. This guarantees that you consume older meals first and assists you in monitoring freshness.
8. **Include Snacks**: Don't forget to prep healthy snacks in addition to main meals. Portion out nuts, cut up fruits and vegetables, and prepare items like hummus or yogurt parfaits. Having ready-to-eat snacks can help you avoid unhealthy options.

Sample Weekly Menus

To help you get started with meal prep, here are two sample weekly menus that align with Dr. Now's dietary principles. These menus provide a variety of nutrient-dense, balanced meals that are easy to prepare in advance.

Sample Menu 1

Monday

- **Breakfast**: Greek yogurt with fresh berries and a sprinkle of chia seeds.
- **Lunch**: Mixed greens, cucumber, cherry tomatoes, and vinaigrette dressing paired with grilled chicken salad.
- **Dinner**: Steamed broccoli and baked salmon with quinoa
- **Snack**: Almond butter on sliced apples.

Tuesday

- **Breakfast**: Overnight oats with almond milk, banana slices, and a drizzle of honey.
- **Lunch**: Turkey and avocado wrap with whole grain tortilla and a side of baby carrots.
- **Dinner**: Brown rice, snap peas, and bell peppers combined with stir-fried tofu.
- **Snack**: Hummus with sliced bell peppers and celery sticks.

Wednesday

- **Breakfast**: Smoothie made with almond milk, protein powder, frozen berries, and spinach.
- **Lunch**: Whole grain bread alongside lentil soup.
- **Dinner**: Grilled shrimp with couscous and roasted asparagus.
- **Snack**: Greek yogurt with a handful of mixed nuts.

Thursday

- **Breakfast**: Toasted whole grain bread with scrambled eggs with spinach.

- **Lunch**: Chickpea salad with tomatoes, cucumbers, feta cheese, and olive oil dressing.
- **Dinner**: Baked chicken breast with sweet potato and green beans.
- **Snack**: Cottage cheese with pineapple chunks.

Friday

- **Breakfast**: Avocado toast with a poached egg on whole grain bread.
- **Lunch**: Bowl of quinoa and black beans with salsa, avocado, and corn.
- **Dinner**: Spaghetti squash with marinara sauce and a side salad.
- **Snack**: Sliced cucumber with tzatziki sauce.

Saturday

- **Breakfast**: Protein pancakes with fresh strawberries and a dollop of Greek yogurt.
- **Lunch**: Tuna salad with mixed greens, cherry tomatoes, and olive oil dressing.
- **Dinner**: Turkey meatballs with whole grain pasta and a side of roasted Brussels sprouts.
- **Snack**: Mixed berry smoothie.

Sunday

- **Breakfast**: Chia pudding with almond milk, topped with blueberries and sliced almonds.
- **Lunch**: Grilled vegetable wrap with hummus and a whole grain tortilla.
- **Dinner**: Beef stir-fry with broccoli, bell peppers, and brown rice.
- **Snack**: Air-popped popcorn.

EXERCISE AND DIET

Importance of Physical Activity in Weight Loss

Physical activity plays a pivotal role in weight loss and overall health. While diet alone can facilitate weight loss, integrating regular exercise amplifies these efforts, leading to more sustainable and holistic health improvements. Exercise helps to burn calories, increase metabolism, and build lean muscle mass, which in turn enhances the body's ability to burn fat. Moreover, physical activity offers numerous psychological benefits, including reduced stress, improved mood, and better sleep, all of which are crucial for maintaining a healthy lifestyle.

Exercise also has profound effects on cardiovascular health, reducing the risk of heart disease, hypertension, and stroke. For individuals struggling with obesity, incorporating physical activity can lead to significant improvements in mobility, joint health, and overall physical function. It's important to remember that the goal is not only to lose weight but to improve overall well-being and quality of life.

Types of Exercises Recommended for Limited Mobility

Many individuals with obesity or related health conditions may find traditional forms of exercise challenging or even daunting. However, it's essential to recognize that exercise can be adapted to fit any fitness level or physical limitation. Here are some types of exercises recommended for those with limited mobility:

1. **Chair Exercises**: These exercises can be performed while seated, making them ideal for individuals with limited mobility or balance issues. Examples include seated leg lifts, arm raises, and chair marching.
2. **Water Aerobics**: Working out in the water offers resistance that promotes strength development while easing the strain on joints and muscles. Water aerobics can be an excellent option for those with arthritis or joint pain.
3. **Stretching and Flexibility Exercises**: Stretching helps improve flexibility, reduce muscle tension, and prevent injuries. Gentle yoga or tai chi can enhance flexibility and promote relaxation.
4. **Resistance Band Exercises**: Resistance bands are versatile tools that can help build muscle strength without the need for heavy weights. They can be used to perform a variety of exercises that target different muscle groups.
5. **Walking**: For those who can manage it, walking is one of the simplest and most effective forms of exercise. It can be done at a pace that suits the individual and gradually increased as endurance improves.
6. **Cycling**: Stationary bikes, particularly recumbent bikes, provide a low-impact cardiovascular workout that can be adjusted to different intensity levels.

How to Integrate Exercise into Daily Routine

Incorporating exercise into your daily routine doesn't have to be overwhelming. Here are some practical tips to help you make physical activity a regular part of your life:

1. **Start Small:** Take it slow and easy at first. Aim for 10 to 15 minutes a day of moderate-length physical activity. Gradually increase the duration and intensity as your fitness level improves.
2. **Set Realistic Goals**: To stay motivated, set realistic fitness goals. Celebrate small milestones to build confidence and maintain momentum.
3. **Create a Schedule**: Just like with any other significant activity, schedule your workouts. Set aside specific times each day for exercise, and stick to the schedule as consistently as possible.

4. **Make It Enjoyable**: Choose activities that you enjoy to make exercise something you look forward to. Whether it's dancing, swimming, or gardening, find what brings you joy and incorporate it into your routine.

5. **Incorporate Movement into Daily Tasks**: Look for opportunities to be active throughout the day. Take the stairs instead of the elevator, walk or cycle for short errands, or do some stretching during TV commercials.

6. **Seek Support**: Engage with a fitness buddy or join a group exercise class. Having social support can enhance motivation and accountability.

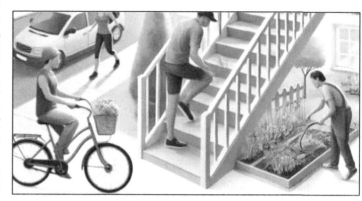

7. **Listen to Your Body**: Observe the way that exercise affects your body. Rest when needed and avoid pushing yourself too hard, especially in the beginning.

FINAL REFLECTIONS ON DR. NOW'S METHOD

Dr. Younan Nowzaradan's method is more than a weight loss regimen; it is a holistic approach to health and well-being. His blend of medical expertise, compassionate care, and unwavering honesty provides a blueprint for individuals struggling with obesity. Dr. Now's success lies in his ability to empower patients, fostering a sense of accountability and self-efficacy. By emphasizing realistic goals, balanced nutrition, and consistent support, he offers a sustainable path to lasting health improvements. His approach transcends the operating room, imparting invaluable lessons on discipline, perseverance, and self-respect.

Call to Action: Starting Your Own Health Journey

Now is the time to take control of your health journey. Embrace the principles outlined in this book, inspired by Dr. Now's proven methods. Begin by setting realistic, achievable goals and commit to making small, incremental changes to your diet and lifestyle. Utilize the recipes and strategies provided to create a balanced, nutritious eating plan. Remember, the journey to better health is a marathon, not a sprint. Stay patient, stay motivated, and seek support when needed. Your transformation starts today. Let Dr. Now's philosophy guide you toward a healthier, happier future. The scale does not lie, and neither should you—embrace this truth and embark on your path to wellness.

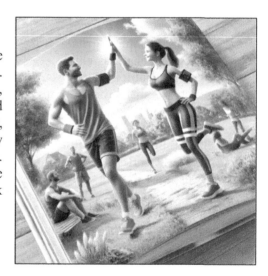

RECIPES

These culinary creations are crafted to help you on your journey to better health, providing you with the tools to make lasting changes in your diet and lifestyle. Whether you're just starting your weight loss journey or looking to maintain a healthy lifestyle, these recipes are designed with your goals in mind.

Eating healthy doesn't mean sacrificing flavor or enjoyment. In fact, the recipes in this book prove that nutritious meals can be both satisfying and delicious. By focusing on whole, natural ingredients and mindful preparation techniques, you'll discover a new appreciation for the food you eat and the benefits it brings to your body.

The Philosophy Behind the Recipes

Each recipe in this collection is inspired by the principles of Dr. Nowzaradan, a pioneer in the field of bariatric surgery and a champion for those battling obesity. His approach emphasizes:

- **Balanced Nutrition**: Ensuring a proper balance of proteins, fats, and carbohydrates to support overall health and well-being.
- **Calorie Control**: Keeping daily caloric intake around 1200 calories to promote steady, sustainable weight loss.
- **Whole Foods**: Focusing on natural, unprocessed ingredients to maximize nutrient intake and minimize empty calories.
- **Flavorful Eating**: Using herbs, spices, and creative combinations to enhance the taste and enjoyment of every meal.

How to Use This Book

This book is divided into sections for breakfasts, main dishes, side dishes, snacks, and desserts. To assist you in keeping track of your consumption and making wise decisions, each dish contains comprehensive nutritional information. The recipes are designed to be simple and accessible, with clear instructions that make preparation a breeze.

As you explore these recipes, remember that variety is key to maintaining interest and excitement in your diet. Feel free to mix and match dishes to suit your tastes and preferences, and don't hesitate to experiment with ingredient substitutions to keep things fresh and enjoyable.

A Journey to Better Health

Embarking on a journey to better health is a personal and rewarding experience. These recipes are more than just meals; they are stepping stones on your path to a healthier, happier life. Embrace the process, celebrate your progress, and enjoy every bite along the way. Remember, this is not just a diet—it's a lifestyle change that will empower you to achieve and maintain your health goals.

BREAKFASTS

Greek Yogurt with Berries and Honey

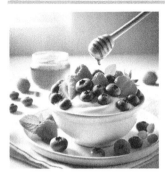

Number of servings: 1
Preparation time: 5 minutes

Ingredients:

- 1 cup Greek yogurt (low-fat)
- 1/2 cup of mixed berries (strawberries, raspberries, and blueberries)
- 1 tbsp honey

Directions:

1. In a bowl, add the Greek yogurt.
2. Top with mixed berries.
3. Drizzle honey over the berries and yogurt.
4. Stir gently to combine all ingredients.

Nutritional value per serving: Calories: 200, Carbs: 32g, Fiber: 4g, Sugars: 24g, Protein: 14g, Saturated fat: 1g, Unsaturated fat: 0g

Difficulty rating: ★☆☆☆☆

Tips for ingredient variations: Substitute honey with maple syrup or agave nectar for a different flavor profile.

Scrambled Egg Whites with Spinach and Feta

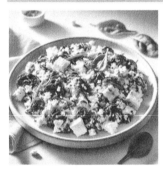

Number of servings: 1
Preparation time: 5 minutes
Cooking time: 5 minutes

Ingredients:

- 4 large egg whites
- 1/2 cup fresh spinach, chopped
- 1 oz feta cheese, crumbled
- 1 tbsp olive oil
- Salt and pepper to taste

Directions:

1. In a nonstick skillet, warm the olive oil over medium heat.
2. Add the chopped spinach and cook until wilted, about 1 minute.
3. Pour in the egg whites and cook, stirring frequently, until the eggs are set but still soft, about 2-3 minutes.
4. Add the crumbled feta cheese and stir to combine.
5. Season with salt and pepper to taste and serve immediately.

Nutritional value per serving: Calories: 150, Carbs: 2g, Fiber: 1g, Sugars: 1g, Protein: 21g, Saturated fat: 3g, Unsaturated fat: 5g

Difficulty rating: ★☆☆☆☆

Tips for ingredient variations: Add diced tomatoes or mushrooms for additional flavor and nutrients.

Oatmeal with Almond Milk, Blueberries, and Chia Seeds

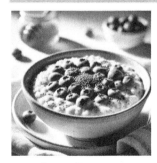

Number of servings: 1
Preparation time: 5 minutes
Cooking time: 5 minutes

Ingredients:

- 1/2 cup rolled oats
- 1 cup almond milk (unsweetened)
- 1/2 cup blueberries
- 1 tbsp chia seeds
- 1 tsp honey (optional)

Directions:

1. In a small pot, bring the almond milk to a boil.
2. Stir in the rolled oats and reduce the heat to a simmer. Cook for about 5 minutes, stirring occasionally, until the oats are soft and the mixture is creamy.
3. Stir in the chia seeds after removing from the heat.
4. Top with blueberries and drizzle with honey if desired.
5. Serve warm.

Nutritional value per serving: Calories: 220, Carbs: 38g, Fiber: 8g, Sugars: 9g, Protein: 6g, Saturated fat: 0g, Unsaturated fat: 4g

Difficulty rating: ★☆☆☆☆

Tips for ingredient variations: Substitute blueberries with your favorite fruit such as strawberries, raspberries, or sliced bananas.

Protein Smoothie (Spinach, Banana, Almond Milk, Protein Powder)

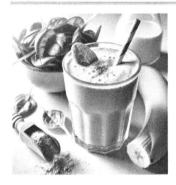

Number of servings: 1

Preparation time: 5 minutes

Ingredients:

- 1 cup fresh spinach
- 1 medium banana
- 1 cup almond milk (unsweetened)
- 1 scoop protein powder (vanilla or unflavored)
- 1/2 cup ice (optional)

Directions:

1. Combine spinach, banana, almond milk, and protein powder in a blender.
2. Blend until smooth.
3. Add ice if desired and blend again until the ice is crushed and the smoothie is creamy.
4. Pour into a glass and serve immediately.

Nutritional value per serving:
Calories: 250, Carbs: 30g, Fiber: 4g, Sugars: 14g, Protein: 20g, Saturated fat: 1g, Unsaturated fat: 2g

Difficulty rating: ★☆☆☆

Tips for ingredient variations:
Add a tablespoon of chia seeds or flax seeds for extra fiber and nutrients.

Whole Wheat Toast with Avocado and Tomato

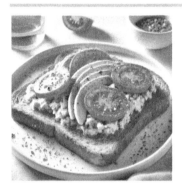

Number of servings: 1

Preparation time: 5 minutes

Ingredients:

- 1 slice whole wheat bread
- 1/2 avocado, mashed
- 1 small tomato, sliced
- Salt and pepper to taste
- Optional: a pinch of red pepper flakes or a drizzle of olive oil

Directions:

1. Toast the whole wheat bread to your desired level of crispiness.
2. Over the toast, equally distribute the mashed avocado.
3. Arrange the tomato slices on top of the avocado.
4. Season with salt and pepper to taste.
5. Add red pepper flakes or a drizzle of olive oil if desired.

Nutritional value per serving:
Calories: 200, Carbs: 22g, Fiber: 8g, Sugars: 2g, Protein: 5g, Saturated fat: 2g, Unsaturated fat: 10g

Difficulty rating: ★☆☆☆

Tips for ingredient variations:
Add a squeeze of lemon juice for a fresh, zesty flavor.

Cottage Cheese with Pineapple and Almonds

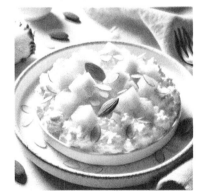

Number of servings: 1

Preparation time: 5 minutes

Ingredients:

- 1/2 cup low-fat cottage cheese
- 1/2 cup pineapple chunks (fresh or canned in juice, drained)
- 1 tbsp sliced almonds

Directions:

1. Place the cottage cheese in a bowl.
2. Top with pineapple chunks.
3. Sprinkle sliced almonds over the top.
4. Serve immediately.

Nutritional value per serving:
Calories: 180, Carbs: 14g, Fiber: 2g, Sugars: 11g, Protein: 14g, Saturated fat: 1g, Unsaturated fat: 4g

Difficulty rating: ★☆☆☆

Tips for ingredient variations:
Substitute pineapple with your favorite fruit such as peaches or berries.

Boiled Eggs and Sliced Avocado

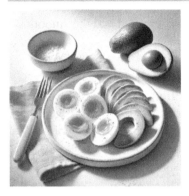

Number of servings: 1
Preparation time: 5 minutes
Cooking time: 10 minutes

Ingredients:

- 2 large eggs
- 1/2 avocado, sliced
- Salt and pepper to taste

Directions:

1. Place the eggs in a pot and cover with water. Bring to a boil.
2. Once boiling, reduce heat to a simmer and cook for 10 minutes.
3. Remove eggs from water and let cool. Peel the eggs.
4. Slice the eggs and avocado.
5. Arrange on a plate and season with salt and pepper to taste.
6. Serve immediately.

Nutritional value per serving: Calories: 200, Carbs: 6g, Fiber: 5g, Sugars: 1g, Protein: 12g, Saturated fat: 3g, Unsaturated fat: 12g

Difficulty rating: ★☆☆☆☆

Tips for ingredient variations: Add a sprinkle of paprika or chili powder for extra flavor.

Apple Slices with Almond Butter and Cinnamon

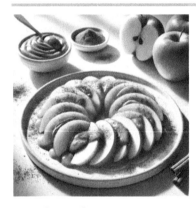

Number of servings: 1
Preparation time: 5 minutes

Ingredients:

- 1 medium apple, sliced
- 1 tbsp almond butter
- 1/2 tsp ground cinnamon

Directions:

1. Core and slice the apple.
2. Arrange apple slices on a plate.
3. Drizzle or spread the almond butter over the apple slices.
4. Sprinkle ground cinnamon on top.
5. Serve immediately.

Nutritional value per serving: Calories: 220, Carbs: 29g, Fiber: 6g, Sugars: 19g, Protein: 4g, Saturated fat: 1g, Unsaturated fat: 8g

Difficulty rating: ★☆☆☆☆

Tips for ingredient variations: Use peanut butter or cashew butter as an alternative to almond butter.

Vegetable Omelette (Egg Whites, Bell Peppers, Onions, Mushrooms)

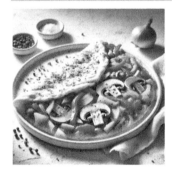

Number of servings: 1
Preparation time: 5 minutes
Cooking time: 5 minutes

Ingredients:

- 4 large egg whites
- 1/4 cup bell peppers, diced
- 1/4 cup onions, diced
- 1/4 cup mushrooms, sliced
- 1 tbsp olive oil
- Salt and pepper to taste

Directions:

1. In a nonstick skillet, heat the olive oil over medium heat.
2. Add bell peppers, onions, and mushrooms to the skillet and cook until vegetables are tender, about 3 minutes.
3. Pour the egg whites over the vegetables and cook until the egg whites are set, about 2-3 minutes.
4. Season with salt and pepper to taste and fold the omelette in half.
5. Serve hot.

Nutritional value per serving: Calories: 200, Carbs: 8g, Fiber: 2g, Sugars: 4g, Protein: 20g, Saturated fat: 1g, Unsaturated fat: 7g

Difficulty rating: ★☆☆☆☆

Tips for ingredient variations: Add a handful of spinach or diced tomatoes for extra flavor and nutrients.

Low-Fat Cheese and Turkey Bacon

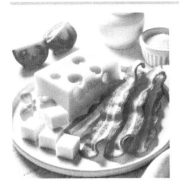

Number of servings: 1
Preparation time: 5 minutes
Cooking time: 5 minutes

Ingredients:

- 2 slices of turkey bacon
- 1 oz low-fat cheese (cheddar, mozzarella, or your choice)

Directions:

1. Heat a non-stick skillet over medium heat.
2. Cook the turkey bacon until crispy, about 2-3 minutes per side.
3. Serve with low-fat cheese on the side.

Nutritional value per serving:
Calories: 200, Carbs: 1g, Fiber: 0g, Sugars: 0g, Protein: 20g, Saturated fat: 5g, Unsaturated fat: 5g

Difficulty rating: ★☆☆☆☆

Tips for ingredient variations:
Pair with a slice of whole grain toast for additional fiber and nutrients.

Chia Seed Pudding with Almond Milk, Strawberries, and Nuts

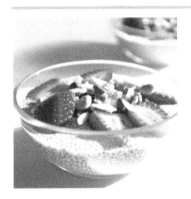

Number of servings: 1
Preparation time: 5 minutes (plus overnight refrigeration)

Ingredients:

- 1/4 cup chia seeds
- 1 cup almond milk (unsweetened)
- 1/2 cup strawberries, sliced
- 1 tbsp mixed nuts, chopped
- 1 tsp honey (optional)

Directions:

1. In a bowl, mix chia seeds and almond milk together.
2. Make sure the chia seeds are dispersed evenly by giving it a good stir.
3. Refrigerate, covered, for at least 4 hours or overnight.
4. Top with sliced strawberries, chopped nuts, and drizzle with honey if desired before serving.

Nutritional value per serving:
Calories: 230, Carbs: 25g, Fiber: 10g, Sugars: 8g, Protein: 8g, Saturated fat: 1g, Unsaturated fat: 12g

Difficulty rating: ★☆☆☆☆

Tips for ingredient variations: Use your favorite fruits such as blueberries or raspberries for a different flavor profile.

Quinoa Porridge with Almonds and Honey

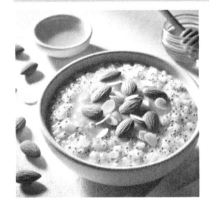

Number of servings: 1
Preparation time: 5 minutes
Cooking time: 15 minutes

Ingredients:

- 1/2 cup quinoa
- 1 cup water
- 1/2 cup almond milk (unsweetened)
- 1 tbsp almonds, sliced
- 1 tsp honey

Directions:

1. Rinse the quinoa under cold water.
2. In a small pot, bring water to a boil.
3. Add quinoa, reduce heat to low, cover, and simmer for about 15 minutes until the quinoa is tender and water is absorbed.
4. Stir in almond milk and cook for another 2-3 minutes.
5. Remove from heat and top with sliced almonds and honey before serving.

Nutritional value per serving:
Calories: 250, Carbs: 42g, Fiber: 5g, Sugars: 8g, Protein: 9g, Saturated fat: 0.5g, Unsaturated fat: 5g

Difficulty rating: ★☆☆☆☆

Tips for ingredient variations:
Add a pinch of cinnamon or nutmeg for additional flavor.

Smoothie Bowl (Berries, Spinach, Almond Milk, Protein Powder, Granola)

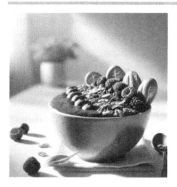

Number of servings: 1
Preparation time: 5 minutes

Ingredients:

- 1/2 cup of mixed berries (strawberries, raspberries, and blueberries)
- 1/2 cup spinach
- 1 cup almond milk (unsweetened)
- 1 scoop protein powder (vanilla or your choice)
- 1/4 cup granola

Directions:

1. In a blender, combine mixed berries, spinach, almond milk, and protein powder.
2. Blend until smooth and thick.
3. Pour into a bowl and top with granola.
4. Serve immediately.

Nutritional value per serving: Calories: 280, Carbs: 34g, Fiber: 8g, Sugars: 16g, Protein: 20g, Saturated fat: 1g, Unsaturated fat: 10g

Difficulty rating: ★☆☆☆☆

Tips for ingredient variations: Add a tablespoon of nut butter or chia seeds for extra protein and healthy fats.

Breakfast Burrito (Egg Whites, Spinach, Whole Wheat Tortilla, Salsa)

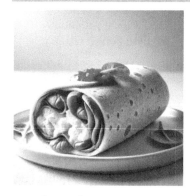

Number of servings: 1
Preparation time: 5 minutes
Cooking time: 5 minutes

Ingredients:

- 4 large egg whites
- 1/2 cup fresh spinach, chopped
- 1 whole wheat tortilla
- 2 tbsp salsa
- 1 tbsp olive oil
- Salt and pepper to taste

Directions:

1. In a nonstick skillet, heat the olive oil over medium heat.
2. Add the chopped spinach and cook until wilted, about 1 minute.
3. Pour in the egg whites and cook, stirring frequently, until the eggs are set but still soft, about 2-3 minutes.
4. Season with salt and pepper to taste.
5. Place the cooked egg whites and spinach in the center of the whole wheat tortilla.
6. Top with salsa and roll up the tortilla to form a burrito.
7. Serve immediately.

Nutritional value per serving: Calories: 250, Carbs: 30g, Fiber: 5g, Sugars: 2g, Protein: 18g, Saturated fat: 1g, Unsaturated fat: 7g

Difficulty rating: ★☆☆☆☆

Tips for ingredient variations: Add black beans or avocado slices for extra flavor and nutrients.

Low-Fat Greek Yogurt with Granola and Berries

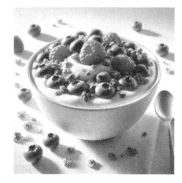

Number of servings: 1
Preparation time: 5 minutes

Ingredients:

- 1 cup low-fat Greek yogurt
- 1/4 cup granola
- 1/2 cup of mixed berries (strawberries, raspberries, and blueberries)

Directions:

1. In a bowl, add the Greek yogurt.
2. Top with granola.
3. Add mixed berries on top of the granola.
4. Stir gently to combine all ingredients.

Nutritional value per serving: Calories: 220, Carbs: 34g, Fiber: 5g, Sugars: 20g, Protein: 12g, Saturated fat: 1g, Unsaturated fat: 4g

Difficulty rating: ★☆☆☆☆

Tips for ingredient variations: Use different types of granola or add a drizzle of honey for extra sweetness.

Pumpkin Spice Oatmeal with Walnuts

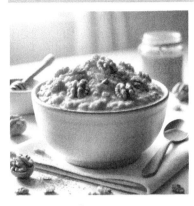

Number of servings: 1

Preparation time: 5 minutes

Cooking time: 5 minutes

Ingredients:

- 1/2 cup rolled oats
- 1 cup almond milk (unsweetened)
- 2 Tbsp of pureed pumpkin
- 1/2 tsp pumpkin spice
- 1 tbsp walnuts, chopped
- 1 tsp honey (optional)

Directions:

1. In a small pot, bring the almond milk to a boil.
2. Stir in the rolled oats and reduce the heat to a simmer. Cook for about 5 minutes, stirring occasionally, until the oats are soft and the mixture is creamy.
3. Stir in the pumpkin puree and pumpkin spice until well combined.
4. Top with chopped walnuts and drizzle with honey if desired.
5. Serve warm.

Nutritional value per serving: Calories: 220, Carbs: 34g, Fiber: 5g, Sugars: 8g, Protein: 6g, Saturated fat: 0g, Unsaturated fat: 4g

Difficulty rating: ★☆☆☆☆

Tips for ingredient variations: Substitute walnuts with pecans or almonds for a different nutty flavor.

Banana Protein Pancakes with Maple Syrup

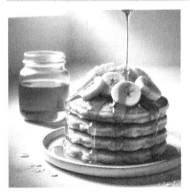

Number of servings: 1

Preparation time: 5 minutes

Cooking time: 10 minutes

Ingredients:

- 1 ripe banana, mashed
- 2 large egg whites
- 1/4 cup rolled oats
- 1/2 scoop vanilla protein powder
- 1/2 tsp baking powder
- 1/4 tsp cinnamon
- 1 tbsp maple syrup

Directions:

1. In a mixing bowl, combine the mashed banana, egg whites, rolled oats, protein powder, baking powder, and cinnamon. Mix until well combined.
2. Coat a nonstick skillet with cooking spray and heat it over medium heat.
3. Pour small portions of the batter onto the skillet to form pancakes.
4. Cook for 2 to 3 minutes on each side, or until bubbles appear on the surface, then turn and continue cooking until both sides are golden brown.
5. Serve the pancakes warm, drizzled with maple syrup.

Nutritional value per serving: Calories: 250, Carbs: 40g, Fiber: 5g, Sugars: 14g, Protein: 14g, Saturated fat: 0g, Unsaturated fat: 2g

Difficulty rating: ★★☆☆☆

Tips for ingredient variations: Add a handful of blueberries or chocolate chips to the batter for extra flavor.

Tomato and Avocado Salad with Olive Oil

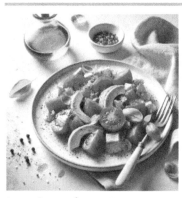

Number of servings: 1
Preparation time: 5 minutes

Ingredients:

- 1 medium tomato, diced
- 1/2 avocado, diced
- 1 tbsp olive oil
- Salt and pepper to taste
- Fresh basil or cilantro (optional)

Directions:

1. In a bowl, combine the diced tomato and avocado.
2. Drizzle with olive oil.
3. Season with salt and pepper to taste.
4. Garnish with fresh basil or cilantro if desired.
5. Serve immediately.

Nutritional value per serving: Calories: 200, Carbs: 10g, Fiber: 7g, Sugars: 2g, Protein: 2g, Saturated fat: 2g, Unsaturated fat: 14g

Difficulty rating: ★☆☆☆

Tips for ingredient variations: Add a squeeze of lime juice or a sprinkle of feta cheese for additional flavor.

Spinach and Mushroom Frittata with Cheese

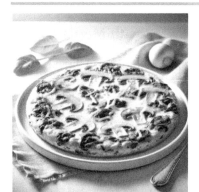

Number of servings: 1
Preparation time: 10 minutes
Cooking time: 10 minutes

Ingredients:

- 3 large egg whites
- 1/4 cup fresh spinach, chopped
- 1/4 cup mushrooms, sliced
- 1/4 cup low-fat cheese, shredded
- 1 tbsp olive oil
- Salt and pepper to taste

Directions:

1. Preheat the oven to 375°F (190°C).
2. In an oven-safe skillet, heat the olive oil over medium heat.
3. Add the mushrooms and spinach, cooking until the spinach is wilted and the mushrooms are tender, about 3-4 minutes.
4. Whisk the egg whites in a bowl with a small amount of salt and pepper.
5. Pour the egg mixture over the vegetables in the skillet. Sprinkle the shredded cheese on top.
6. After transferring the pan to the oven, preheat it and bake it for 5 to 7 minutes, or until the cheese has melted and the eggs are set.
7. Remove from the oven and let it cool for a minute before serving.

Nutritional value per serving: Calories: 220, Carbs: 4g, Fiber: 1g, Sugars: 2g, Protein: 18g, Saturated fat: 3g, Unsaturated fat: 8g

Difficulty rating: ★★☆☆

Tips for ingredient variations: Add diced bell peppers or onions for extra flavor and nutrients.

Berry and Almond Smoothie

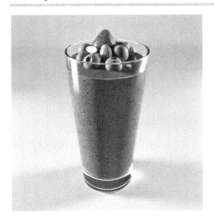

Number of servings: 1
Preparation time: 5 minutes

Ingredients:

- 1/2 cup almond milk (unsweetened)
- 1/2 cup of mixed berries (strawberries, raspberries, and blueberries)
- 1/4 cup Greek yogurt (low-fat)
- 1 tbsp almond butter
- 1 tsp honey (optional)
- 1/2 cup ice cubes

Directions:

1. Combine all ingredients in a blender.
2. Blend until smooth and creamy.
3. Pour into a glass and serve immediately.

Nutritional value per serving: Calories: 230, Carbs: 26g, Fiber: 6g, Sugars: 16g, Protein: 9g, Saturated fat: 0.5g, Unsaturated fat: 8g

Difficulty rating: ★☆☆☆☆

Tips for ingredient variations: Add a scoop of protein powder for an extra protein boost or substitute almond butter with peanut butter.

Peanut Butter Banana Toast with Chia Seeds

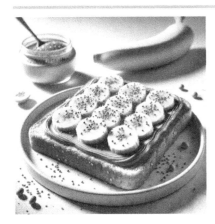

Number of servings: 1
Preparation time: 5 minutes

Ingredients:

- 1 slice whole wheat bread
- 1 tbsp peanut butter (natural, unsweetened)
- 1/2 banana, sliced
- 1 tsp chia seeds

Directions:

1. Toast the slice of whole wheat bread until golden brown.
2. Over the bread, evenly distribute the peanut butter.
3. Arrange the banana slices on top of the peanut butter.
4. Sprinkle chia seeds over the banana slices.
5. Serve immediately.

Nutritional value per serving: Calories: 220, Carbs: 30g, Fiber: 5g, Sugars: 9g, Protein: 6g, Saturated fat: 1g, Unsaturated fat: 8g

Difficulty rating: ★☆☆☆☆

Tips for ingredient variations: For a different flavor, try almond or cashew butter in instead of peanut butter.

Mixed Fruit Salad with Greek Yogurt

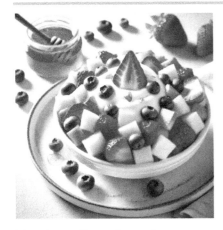

Number of servings: 1
Preparation time: 10 minutes

Ingredients:

- 1/2 cup Greek yogurt (low-fat)
- 1/4 cup strawberries, sliced
- 1/4 cup blueberries
- 1/4 cup pineapple chunks
- 1/4 cup apple, diced
- 1 tsp honey (optional)

Directions:

1. In a bowl, mix all the fruits together.
2. Spoon the Greek yogurt over the mixed fruits.
3. Drizzle honey on top if desired.
4. Stir gently to combine all ingredients and serve immediately.

Nutritional value per serving: Calories: 200, Carbs: 38g, Fiber: 4g, Sugars: 27g, Protein: 10g, Saturated fat: 1g, Unsaturated fat: 0g

Difficulty rating: ★☆☆☆☆

Tips for ingredient variations: Add a sprinkle of granola for a crunchy texture.

Zucchini Bread with Cream Cheese

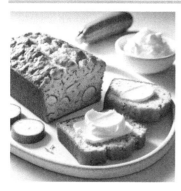

Number of servings: 1
Preparation time: 10 minutes
Cooking time: 40 minutes

Ingredients:

- 1 cup grated zucchini
- 1 cup whole wheat flour
- 1/4 cup applesauce (unsweetened)
- 1/4 cup honey
- 1 egg
- 1 tsp vanilla extract
- 1 tsp baking soda
- 1/2 tsp ground cinnamon
- 1/4 tsp salt
- 1/4 cup low-fat cream cheese, softened

Directions:

1. Preheat the oven to 350°F (175°C). Grease a loaf pan or line it with parchment paper.
2. In a large bowl, combine the grated zucchini, applesauce, honey, egg, and vanilla extract.
3. In a separate bowl, mix the whole wheat flour, baking soda, ground cinnamon, and salt.
4. Stirring until just blended, gradually add the dry ingredients to the wet components.
5. Pour the batter into the prepared loaf pan and bake for 35-40 minutes, or until a toothpick inserted into the center comes out clean.
6. Allow the bread to cool completely in the pan before removing and slicing.
7. Spread the softened cream cheese on a slice of zucchini bread before serving.

Nutritional value per serving: Calories: 220, Carbs: 35g, Fiber: 4g, Sugars: 15g, Protein: 6g, Saturated fat: 2g, Unsaturated fat: 3g

Difficulty rating: ★★☆☆☆

Tips for ingredient variations: Add chopped nuts or raisins for added texture and flavor.

Almond Butter and Banana Smoothie with Protein Powder

Number of servings: 1
Preparation time: 5 minutes

Ingredients:

- 1 medium banana
- 1 tbsp almond butter
- 1 scoop vanilla protein powder
- 1 cup almond milk (unsweetened)
- 1/2 cup ice cubes

Directions:

1. In blender, combine all ingredients.
2. Blend on high until creamy and smooth.
3. Transfer into a glass and serve right away.

Nutritional value per serving: Calories: 250, Carbs: 34g, Fiber: 5g, Sugars: 16g, Protein: 20g, Saturated fat: 0.5g, Unsaturated fat: 5g

Difficulty rating: ★☆☆☆☆

Tips for ingredient variations: Add a handful of spinach for extra nutrients without altering the flavor.

Egg Muffins with Veggies and Cheese

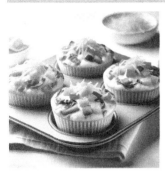

Number of servings: 6 muffins
Preparation time: 10 minutes
Cooking time: 20 minutes

Ingredients:

- 6 large eggs
- 1/2 cup of bell peppers, chopped
- 1/2 cup chopped spinach
- 1/4 cup diced onions
- 1/4 cup shredded cheese of your choice
- Salt and pepper to taste
- Cooking spray

Directions:

1. Preheat the oven to 350°F (175°C).
2. Spray a muffin tin with cooking spray.
3. In a bowl, whisk the eggs and season with salt and pepper.
4. To the egg mixture, add the chopped onions, diced bell peppers, and chopped spinach.
5. Evenly pour the mixture into the muffin pan.
6. Top each muffin with a small amount of shredded cheese.
7. Bake for 20 minutes or until the egg muffins are set and lightly browned on top.
8. Take out of the oven and let it to cool down for several minutes before serving.

Nutritional value per serving (2 muffins): Calories: 200, Carbs: 4g, Fiber: 1g, Sugars: 2g, Protein: 15g, Saturated fat: 3g, Unsaturated fat: 5g

Difficulty rating: ★☆☆☆☆

Tips for ingredient variations: Use different vegetables such as mushrooms, tomatoes, or zucchini to change the flavor profile.

Tropical Smoothie (Mango, Pineapple, Coconut Milk, Chia Seeds)

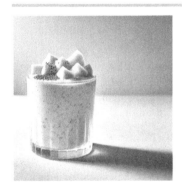

Number of servings: 1
Preparation time: 5 minutes

Ingredients:

- 1/2 cup frozen mango chunks
- 1/2 cup frozen pineapple chunks
- 1 cup coconut milk (unsweetened)
- 1 tbsp chia seeds
- 1/2 cup ice cubes

Directions:

1. Combine all ingredients in a blender.
2. Blend on high until smooth and creamy.
3. Pour into a glass and serve immediately.

Nutritional value per serving: Calories: 230, Carbs: 36g, Fiber: 8g, Sugars: 24g, Protein: 4g, Saturated fat: 3g, Unsaturated fat: 2g

Difficulty rating: ★☆☆☆☆

Tips for ingredient variations: Add a handful of spinach for extra nutrients without altering the flavor.

Oatmeal with Chia Seeds, Fresh Berries, and Almonds

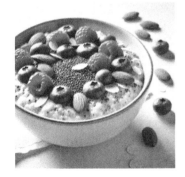

Number of servings: 1
Preparation time: 5 minutes
Cooking time: 5 minutes

Ingredients:

- 1/2 cup rolled oats
- 1 cup almond milk (unsweetened)
- 1/2 cup mixed fresh berries (blueberries, strawberries, raspberries)
- 1 tbsp chia seeds
- 1 tbsp sliced almonds
- 1 tsp honey (optional)

Directions:

1. In a small pot, bring the almond milk to a boil.
2. Stir in the rolled oats and reduce the heat to a simmer. Cook for about 5 minutes, stirring occasionally, until the oats are soft and the mixture is creamy.
3. Stir in the chia seeds after removing from the heat.
4. Top with mixed berries and sliced almonds.
5. Drizzle with honey if desired.
6. Serve warm.

Nutritional value per serving: Calories: 230, Carbs: 36g, Fiber: 8g, Sugars: 12g, Protein: 7g, Saturated fat: 0.5g, Unsaturated fat: 5g

Difficulty rating: ★☆☆☆☆

Tips for ingredient variations: Substitute berries with your favorite fruit such as sliced bananas, peaches, or apples.

Turkey Sausage and Veggie Scramble

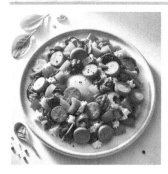

Number of servings: 1
Preparation time: 5 minutes
Cooking time: 10 minutes

Ingredients:

- 2 turkey sausage links, sliced
- 2 large eggs
- 1/4 cup diced bell peppers
- 1/4 cup diced onions
- 1/4 cup chopped spinach
- 1 tbsp olive oil
- Salt and pepper to taste

Directions:

1. In a nonstick skillet, heat the olive oil over medium heat.
2. Add the sliced turkey sausage and cook until browned, about 3-4 minutes.
3. Add the diced bell peppers and onions, and cook until softened, about 2-3 minutes.
4. Stir in the chopped spinach and cook until wilted, about 1 minute.
5. In a bowl, whisk the eggs and season with salt and pepper.
6. Pour the eggs into the skillet and cook, stirring frequently, until the eggs are set but still soft, about 2-3 minutes.
7. Serve immediately.

Nutritional value per serving: Calories: 250, Carbs: 4g, Fiber: 1g, Sugars: 2g, Protein: 21g, Saturated fat: 3g, Unsaturated fat: 10g

Difficulty rating: ★☆☆☆☆

Tips for ingredient variations: Add diced tomatoes or mushrooms for additional flavor and nutrients.

Ricotta Cheese with Fresh Berries and Honey

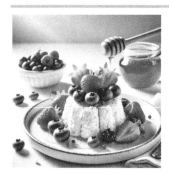

Number of servings: 1
Preparation time: 5 minutes

Ingredients:

- 1/2 cup ricotta cheese (part-skim)
- 1/2 cup fresh mixed berries (blueberries, strawberries, raspberries)
- 1 tsp honey

Directions:

1. Place the ricotta cheese in a serving bowl.
2. Top with the fresh mixed berries.
3. Drizzle honey over the berries and ricotta cheese.
4. Stir gently to combine all ingredients.

Nutritional value per serving: Calories: 200, Carbs: 23g, Fiber: 4g, Sugars: 17g, Protein: 10g, Saturated fat: 3g, Unsaturated fat: 2g

Difficulty rating: ★☆☆☆☆

Tips for ingredient variations: Add a sprinkle of chopped nuts or a dash of cinnamon for added flavor and texture.

Low-Carb Breakfast Wrap (Lettuce, Turkey, Cheese, Avocado)

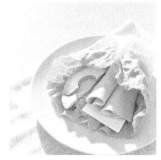

Number of servings: 1
Preparation time: 10 minutes

Ingredients:

- 2 large lettuce leaves (e.g., romaine or iceberg)
- 2 slices deli turkey breast (low sodium)
- 1 slice cheese (e.g., Swiss or cheddar)
- 1/4 avocado, sliced
- 1 tbsp light mayonnaise (optional)
- Salt and pepper to taste

Directions:

1. Lay the lettuce leaves flat on a plate.
2. Place the turkey slices on top of the lettuce leaves.
3. Place the cheese slice over the turkey.
4. Arrange the avocado slices on top of the cheese.
5. If desired, spread a thin layer of light mayonnaise over the avocado slices.
6. Season with salt and pepper to taste.
7. Roll the lettuce leaves tightly to form a wrap. Secure with a toothpick if necessary.
8. Serve immediately.

Nutritional value per serving: Calories: 220, Carbs: 6g, Fiber: 4g, Sugars: 2g, Protein: 14g, Saturated fat: 4g, Unsaturated fat: 7g

Difficulty rating: ★☆☆☆☆

Tips for ingredient variations: Add slices of tomato or cucumber for extra crunch and flavor.

MAIN DISHES

Grilled Chicken Breast with Steamed Broccoli and Quinoa

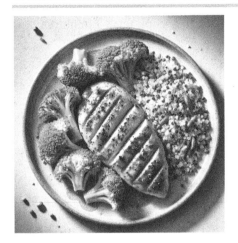

Number of servings: 1
Preparation time: 10 minutes
Cooking time: 20 minutes

Ingredients:

- 1 (4 oz) chicken breast, boneless and skinless
- 1 cup broccoli florets
- 1/2 cup cooked quinoa
- 1 tbsp olive oil
- 1 tsp garlic powder
- Salt and pepper to taste
- 1/2 lemon (optional for garnish)

Directions:

1. Preheat the grill to medium-high heat.
2. Season the chicken breast with olive oil, garlic powder, salt, and pepper.
3. Grill the chicken for 6-7 minutes on each side, or until the internal temperature reaches 165°F (74°C).
4. While the chicken is grilling, steam the broccoli florets until tender, about 5-7 minutes.
5. Serve the grilled chicken breast with steamed broccoli and cooked quinoa on the side.
6. If preferred, garnish with a squeeze of lemon.

Nutritional value per serving: Calories: 350, Carbs: 32g, Fiber: 5g, Sugars: 2g, Protein: 35g, Saturated fat: 2g, Unsaturated fat: 10g

Difficulty rating: ★☆☆☆☆

Tips for ingredient variations: Add a side of mixed greens for extra nutrients.

Baked Salmon with Asparagus and Brown Rice

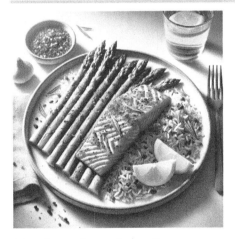

Number of servings: 1
Preparation time: 10 minutes
Cooking time: 20 minutes

Ingredients:

- 1 (4 oz) salmon fillet
- 1 cup asparagus spears, trimmed
- 1/2 cup cooked brown rice
- 1 tbsp olive oil
- 1 tsp lemon zest
- 1 tsp garlic powder
- Salt and pepper to taste

Directions:

1. Preheat the oven to 400°F (200°C).
2. Place the salmon fillet onto a parchment paper-lined baking sheet.
3. Drizzle the salmon and asparagus with olive oil, and season with lemon zest, garlic powder, salt, and pepper.
4. Bake the salmon for 15 to 20 minutes, or until it is cooked through and flake readily when tested with a fork.
5. Serve the baked salmon with asparagus and cooked brown rice on the side.

Nutritional value per serving: Calories: 380, Carbs: 35g, Fiber: 5g, Sugars: 2g, Protein: 28g, Saturated fat: 3g, Unsaturated fat: 15g

Difficulty rating: ★☆☆☆☆

Tips for ingredient variations: Substitute asparagus with green beans or broccoli for variety.

Turkey Meatballs with Zucchini Noodles and Marinara Sauce

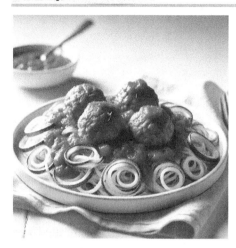

Number of servings: 1
Preparation time: 15 minutes
Cooking time: 20 minutes

Ingredients:

- 4 oz ground turkey
- 1/4 cup breadcrumbs
- 1 egg white
- 1 tbsp grated Parmesan cheese
- 1 tsp Italian seasoning
- 1 medium zucchini, spiralized
- 1/2 cup marinara sauce
- 1 tbsp olive oil
- Salt and pepper to taste

Directions:

1. Preheat the oven to 375°F (190°C).
2. In a bowl, mix the ground turkey, breadcrumbs, egg white, Parmesan cheese, Italian seasoning, salt, and pepper.
3. Shape the mixture into little meatballs and arrange them on a parchment paper-lined baking sheet.
4. Bake the meatballs for 15-20 minutes, or until cooked through and golden brown.
5. Heat the olive oil in a pan over medium heat. Add the zucchini noodles and cook for 2-3 minutes until tender.
6. Heat the marinara sauce in a small pot over medium heat.
7. Serve the turkey meatballs over the zucchini noodles, topped with marinara sauce.

Nutritional value per serving: Calories: 320, Carbs: 22g, Fiber: 5g, Sugars: 7g, Protein: 28g, Saturated fat: 2g, Unsaturated fat: 10g

Difficulty rating: ★☆☆☆☆

Tips for ingredient variations: Add chopped fresh basil or parsley for additional flavor.

Stir-Fried Vegetables with Brown Rice and Tofu

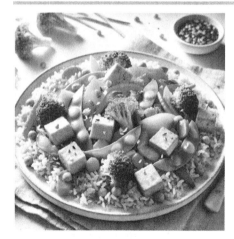

Number of servings: 1
Preparation time: 10 minutes
Cooking time: 15 minutes

Ingredients:

- 4 oz firm tofu, cubed
- One cup of mixed veggies (carrots, snap peas, broccoli, bell peppers)
- 1/2 cup cooked brown rice
- 1 tbsp soy sauce
- 1 tbsp olive oil
- 1 tsp grated ginger
- 1 clove garlic, minced
- Salt and pepper to taste

Directions:

1. In a skillet, heat the olive oil over medium-high heat.
2. Add the cubed tofu and cook until golden brown, about 5-7 minutes. Remove from the skillet and set aside.
3. In the same skillet, add the mixed vegetables, grated ginger, and minced garlic. Stir-fry for 5-7 minutes until the vegetables are tender-crisp.
4. Return the tofu to the skillet and then cover it with the soy sauce. Stir to combine and cook for another 2 minutes.
5. Pour the cooked brown rice over the vegetable stir-fry.

Nutritional value per serving: Calories: 350, Carbs: 40g, Fiber: 8g, Sugars: 6g, Protein: 14g, Saturated fat: 2g, Unsaturated fat: 12g

Difficulty rating: ★☆☆☆☆

Tips for ingredient variations: Add sesame seeds or a splash of sesame oil for an extra layer of flavor.

Quinoa Salad with Chickpeas, Veggies, and Feta

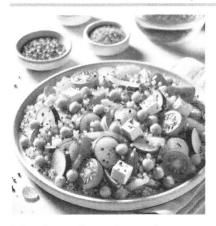

Number of servings: 1
Preparation time: 10 minutes
Cooking time: 15 minutes (for quinoa)

Ingredients:

- 1/2 cup cooked quinoa
- 1/2 cup canned chickpeas, rinsed and drained
- 1/4 cup diced cucumber
- 1/4 cup diced tomatoes
- 1/4 cup diced bell peppers
- 1 oz feta cheese, crumbled
- 1 tbsp olive oil
- 1 tbsp lemon juice
- 1 tsp dried oregano
- Salt and pepper to taste

Directions:

1. In a large bowl, combine the cooked quinoa, chickpeas, cucumber, tomatoes, bell peppers, and feta cheese.
2. In a small bowl, whisk together the olive oil, lemon juice, dried oregano, salt, and pepper.
3. Mix the quinoa mixture with the dressing after pouring it over it.
4. Serve cold or room temperature.

Nutritional value per serving: Calories: 380, Carbs: 45g, Fiber: 9g, Sugars: 6g, Protein: 12g, Saturated fat: 3g, Unsaturated fat: 15g

Difficulty rating: ★☆☆☆☆

Tips for ingredient variations: Add chopped fresh herbs like parsley or mint for extra freshness.

Grilled Shrimp Skewers with Bell Peppers and Couscous

Number of servings: 2
Preparation time: 15 minutes
Cooking time: 10 minutes

Ingredients:

- 12 large shrimp, peeled and deveined
- 1 bell pepper, cut into chunks
- 1 tbsp olive oil
- 1 tsp garlic powder
- 1 tsp paprika
- Salt and pepper to taste
- 1 cup cooked couscous

Directions:

1. Preheat the grill to medium-high heat.
2. In a bowl, toss the shrimp and bell pepper chunks with olive oil, garlic powder, paprika, salt, and pepper.
3. Put the bell peppers and shrimp on skewers.
4. Grill the skewers for about 2-3 minutes on each side, until the shrimp are pink and cooked through.
5. Serve the shrimp skewers over a bed of cooked couscous.

Nutritional value per serving: Calories: 330, Carbs: 34g, Fiber: 4g, Sugars: 2g, Protein: 25g, Saturated fat: 2g, Unsaturated fat: 8g

Difficulty rating: ★★☆☆☆

Tips for ingredient variations: Substitute couscous with quinoa or brown rice for a different grain option.

Spaghetti Squash with Marinara Sauce and Parmesan

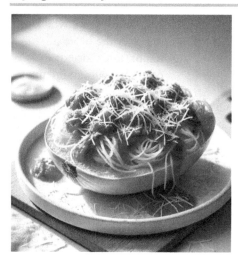

Number of servings: 2
Preparation time: 10 minutes
Cooking time: 40 minutes

Ingredients:

- 1 medium spaghetti squash
- 1 cup marinara sauce (low-sugar)
- 1/4 cup grated Parmesan cheese
- 1 tbsp olive oil
- Salt and pepper to taste

Directions:

1. Preheat the oven to 400°F (200°C).
2. After slicing the spaghetti squash in half lengthwise, remove the seeds.
3. Drizzle the inside of the squash with olive oil and season with salt and pepper.
4. Place the squash halves cut side down on a baking sheet and roast for 30-40 minutes, until the flesh is tender and easily shredded with a fork.
5. While the squash is roasting, heat the marinara sauce in a small pot.
6. Once the squash is cooked, use a fork to scrape out the spaghetti-like strands into a bowl.
7. Toss the squash with marinara sauce and top with grated Parmesan cheese.
8. Serve warm.

Nutritional value per serving:
Calories: 280, Carbs: 28g, Fiber: 6g, Sugars: 10g, Protein: 8g, Saturated fat: 3g, Unsaturated fat: 5g

Difficulty rating: ★★☆☆☆

Tips for ingredient variations:
Add sautéed mushrooms or ground turkey to the marinara sauce for additional protein and flavor.

Chicken and Vegetable Soup with Barley

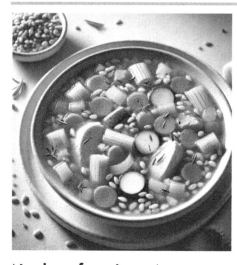

Number of servings: 4
Preparation time: 10 minutes
Cooking time: 30 minutes

Ingredients:

- 1 lb boneless, skinless chicken breast, cubed
- 1 cup barley, uncooked
- 2 carrots, diced
- 2 celery stalks, diced
- 1 onion, chopped
- 1 zucchini, diced
- 8 cups chicken broth (low-sodium)
- 1 tbsp olive oil
- 1 tsp thyme
- 1 tsp rosemary
- Salt and pepper to taste

Directions:

1. In a big pot, heat the olive oil over medium heat.
2. Add the chicken and cook until browned, about 5-7 minutes.
3. After adding the onion, carrots, and celery, simmer for about five minutes, or until the veggies are tender.
4. Stir in the barley and cook for 2 minutes.
5. Add the chicken broth, thyme, rosemary, salt, and pepper. Bring to a boil.
6. Reduce the heat to a simmer and cook for about 20 minutes, until the barley is tender.
7. Cook for a further five minutes after adding the zucchini.
8. Serve hot.

Nutritional value per serving:
Calories: 300, Carbs: 38g, Fiber: 8g, Sugars: 6g, Protein: 25g, Saturated fat: 1g, Unsaturated fat: 4g

Difficulty rating: ★★☆☆☆

Tips for ingredient variations:
Use quinoa or brown rice instead of barley for a gluten-free option.

Turkey and Avocado Lettuce Wraps with Salsa

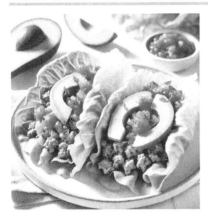

Number of servings: 2
Preparation time: 10 minutes
Cooking time: 10 minutes

Ingredients:

- 1 lb ground turkey
- 1 avocado, sliced
- 1 cup salsa (fresh or store-bought)
- 8 large lettuce leaves (Romaine or Butter lettuce)
- 1 tbsp olive oil
- 1 tsp cumin
- 1 tsp paprika
- Salt and pepper to taste

Directions:

1. Heat the olive oil in a skillet over medium heat.
2. Add the ground turkey, cumin, paprika, salt, and pepper. Cook for 8 to 10 minutes, or until the turkey is browned and cooked through.
3. Lay out the lettuce leaves and fill each with cooked turkey.
4. Top with avocado slices and salsa.
5. Roll up the lettuce wraps and serve immediately.

Nutritional value per serving:
Calories: 280, Carbs: 8g, Fiber: 6g, Sugars: 2g, Protein: 28g, Saturated fat: 3g, Unsaturated fat: 12g

Difficulty rating: ★☆☆☆☆

Tips for ingredient variations: Add diced bell peppers or shredded cheese for extra flavor and texture.

Baked Cod with Lemon, Dill, and Wild Rice

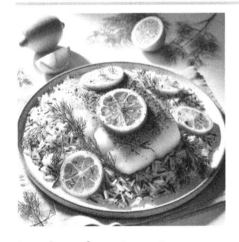

Number of servings: 2
Preparation time: 10 minutes
Cooking time: 20 minutes

Ingredients:

- 2 cod fillets (6 oz each)
- 1 lemon, sliced
- 1 tbsp fresh dill, chopped
- 1 tbsp olive oil
- Salt and pepper to taste
- 1 cup cooked wild rice

Directions:

1. Preheat the oven to 375°F (190°C).
2. Place the cod fillets in a baking dish and drizzle with olive oil.
3. Season the fish with salt and pepper, and top with lemon slices and fresh dill.
4. Bake for 15-20 minutes, until the fish is opaque and flakes easily with a fork.
5. Serve the cod fillets over a bed of cooked wild rice.

Nutritional value per serving:
Calories: 320, Carbs: 36g, Fiber: 4g, Sugars: 1g, Protein: 30g, Saturated fat: 1g, Unsaturated fat: 5g

Difficulty rating: ★☆☆☆☆

Tips for ingredient variations: Add a side of steamed vegetables or a light salad for a complete meal.

Chicken Stir-Fry with Brown Rice and Veggies

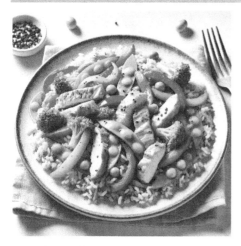

Number of servings: 1
Preparation time: 10 minutes
Cooking time: 15 minutes

Ingredients:

- 4 oz chicken breast, sliced into strips
- 1 cup mixed vegetables (bell peppers, broccoli, snap peas)
- 1/2 cup cooked brown rice
- 1 tbsp soy sauce (low sodium)
- 1 tbsp olive oil
- 1 clove garlic, minced
- 1 tsp fresh ginger, minced
- Salt and pepper to taste

Directions:

1. In a large skillet or wok, heat the olive oil over medium-high heat.
2. Add the minced garlic and ginger, and stir-fry for about 1 minute until fragrant.
3. Add the chicken strips and cook until no longer pink, about 5-7 minutes.
4. Add the mixed vegetables and stir-fry until tender-crisp, about 5 minutes.
5. Stir in the soy sauce and cooked brown rice, and mix until everything is well combined and heated through.
6. Season with salt and pepper to taste, and serve immediately.

Nutritional value per serving: Calories: 380, Carbs: 38g, Fiber: 5g, Sugars: 4g, Protein: 28g, Saturated fat: 1g, Unsaturated fat: 10g

Difficulty rating: ★★☆☆

Tips for ingredient variations: Substitute chicken with shrimp or tofu for a different protein option.

Vegetarian Chili with Quinoa

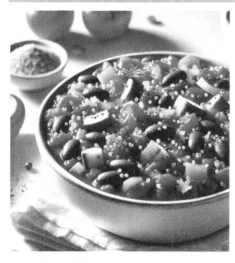

Number of servings: 4
Preparation time: 15 minutes
Cooking time: 30 minutes

Ingredients:

- 1 cup quinoa, rinsed
- 1 tbsp olive oil
- 1 onion, diced
- 2 cloves garlic, minced
- 1 bell pepper, diced
- 1 zucchini, diced
- 1 can (15 oz) black beans, drained and rinsed
- 1 can (15 oz) kidney beans, drained and rinsed
- 1 can (15 oz) diced tomatoes
- 2 cups vegetable broth
- 2 tbsp chili powder
- 1 tsp cumin
- 1 tsp paprika
- Salt and pepper to taste

Directions:

1. Heat the olive oil in a big pot over medium heat. Add the onion and garlic, and cook until softened, about 5 minutes.
2. Add the bell pepper and zucchini, and cook for another 5 minutes.
3. Stir in the quinoa, black beans, kidney beans, diced tomatoes, vegetable broth, chili powder, cumin, and paprika. Bring to a boil.
4. Reduce heat to low, cover, and simmer for 20 minutes, or until the quinoa is cooked and the flavors have melded together.
5. Season with salt and pepper to taste and serve.

Nutritional value per serving: Calories: 330, Carbs: 54g, Fiber: 14g, Sugars: 8g, Protein: 14g, Saturated fat: 1g, Unsaturated fat: 6g

Difficulty rating: ★★☆☆

Tips for ingredient variations: Add corn, carrots, or any other favorite vegetables to enhance the flavor and nutrition.

Stuffed Bell Peppers with Ground Turkey and Brown Rice

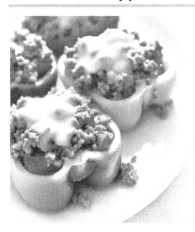

Number of servings: 4
Preparation time: 15 minutes
Cooking time: 45 minutes

Ingredients:

- 4 large bell peppers with the seeds removed and the tops removed
- 1 lb ground turkey
- 1 cup cooked brown rice
- 1 onion, diced
- 1 can (15 oz) diced tomatoes
- 1 cup shredded mozzarella cheese (optional)
- 1 tbsp olive oil
- 2 cloves garlic, minced
- 1 tsp dried oregano
- 1 tsp dried basil
- Salt and pepper to taste

Directions:

1. Preheat the oven to 375°F (190°C).
2. In a large skillet, heat the olive oil over medium heat. Add the onion and garlic, and cook until softened, about 5 minutes.
3. Add the ground turkey and cook until browned, about 7 minutes.
4. Stir in the diced tomatoes, cooked brown rice, oregano, basil, salt, and pepper. Cook for another 5 minutes.
5. Stuff each bell pepper with the turkey mixture, pressing down slightly to fill.
6. Place the stuffed peppers in a baking dish. If using, sprinkle the shredded mozzarella cheese on top.
7. Bake for 30 minutes in a preheated oven, or until the cheese is bubbling and melted and the peppers are soft.
8. Serve hot.

Nutritional value per serving:
Calories: 340, Carbs: 28g, Fiber: 6g, Sugars: 8g, Protein: 28g, Saturated fat: 3g, Unsaturated fat: 10g

Difficulty rating: ★★☆☆☆

Tips for ingredient variations: Substitute ground turkey with ground chicken or beef for a different flavor.

Black Bean and Corn Salad with Avocado

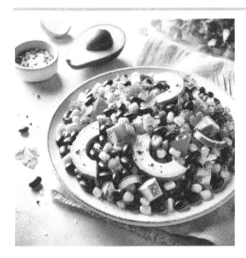

Number of servings: 4
Preparation time: 10 minutes

Ingredients:

- 1 can (15 oz) black beans, drained and rinsed
- 1 cup corn kernels (fresh, frozen, or canned)
- 1 avocado, diced
- 1 red bell pepper, diced
- 1/2 red onion, finely chopped
- 1/4 cup fresh cilantro, chopped
- 2 tbsp olive oil
- 1 lime, juiced
- Salt and pepper to taste

Directions:

1. Combine the black beans, corn, avocado, red onion, red bell pepper, and cilantro in a big bowl.
2. Mix the olive oil, lime juice, salt, and pepper in a small bowl.
3. Drizzle the salad with the dressing and gently toss to mix.
4. To let the flavors mingle, serve right away or chill for up to two hours in the refrigerator.

Nutritional value per serving:
Calories: 300, Carbs: 38g, Fiber: 12g, Sugars: 3g, Protein: 8g, Saturated fat: 2g, Unsaturated fat: 12g

Difficulty rating: ★☆☆☆☆

Tips for ingredient variations: Add diced tomatoes or jalapenos for extra flavor and heat.

Baked Tilapia with Spinach and Sweet Potato

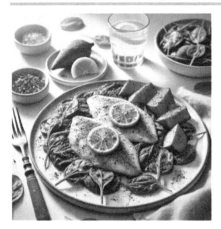

Number of servings: 4
Preparation time: 10 minutes
Cooking time: 20 minutes

Ingredients:

- 4 tilapia fillets
- 2 cups fresh spinach
- 2 medium sweet potatoes, peeled and cubed
- 2 tbsp olive oil
- 1 lemon, sliced
- 2 cloves garlic, minced
- 1 tsp paprika
- Salt and pepper to taste

Directions:

1. Preheat the oven to 400°F (200°C).
2. Place the sweet potato cubes on a baking sheet and drizzle with 1 tbsp olive oil. Season with salt, pepper, and paprika. Toss to coat evenly.
3. Bake the sweet potatoes in the preheated oven for 10 minutes.
4. Meanwhile, heat the remaining 1 tbsp olive oil in a skillet over medium heat. Cook for a minute after adding the minced garlic.
5. Add the spinach to the skillet and cook until wilted, about 2-3 minutes.
6. Remove the baking sheet from the oven and push the sweet potatoes to one side. Place the tilapia fillets on the other side of the baking sheet. Top each fillet with lemon slices.
7. Return the baking sheet to the oven and bake for an additional 10 minutes, or until the tilapia is cooked through and flakes easily with a fork.
8. Serve the tilapia with the roasted sweet potatoes and wilted spinach.

Nutritional value per serving:
Calories: 330, Carbs: 34g, Fiber: 8g, Sugars: 7g, Protein: 28g, Saturated fat: 2g, Unsaturated fat: 12g

Difficulty rating: ★★☆☆☆

Tips for ingredient variations: Substitute tilapia with another white fish like cod or haddock.

Cauliflower Fried Rice with Chicken and Veggies

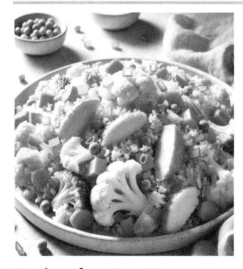

Number of servings: 2
Preparation time: 10 minutes
Cooking time: 15 minutes

Ingredients:

- 1 medium head cauliflower, grated or pulsed in a food processor to resemble rice
- 1 cup cooked chicken breast, diced
- 1 cup mixed vegetables (carrots, peas, bell peppers), diced
- 2 tbsp soy sauce (low sodium)
- 1 tbsp sesame oil
- 2 cloves garlic, minced
- 1 small onion, diced
- 2 eggs, lightly beaten
- 2 green onions, sliced
- Salt and pepper to taste

Directions:

1. Heat sesame oil in a large skillet or wok over medium-high heat.
2. Add garlic and onion, and sauté until fragrant, about 2 minutes.
3. Add mixed vegetables and cook for about 3-4 minutes until tender.
4. Transfer the vegetables to one side of the skillet and then fill the void with the whisked eggs. Scramble the eggs until cooked through.
5. Stir in the grated cauliflower, cooked chicken, and soy sauce. Cook for another 5 minutes, stirring occasionally.
6. Season with salt and pepper to taste.
7. Garnish with sliced green onions before serving.

Nutritional value per serving:
Calories: 340, Carbs: 20g, Fiber: 7g, Sugars: 5g, Protein: 30g, Saturated fat: 2g, Unsaturated fat: 8g

Difficulty rating: ★★☆☆☆

Tips for ingredient variations: Substitute chicken with shrimp or tofu for a different protein option.

Lentil Soup with Spinach and Carrots

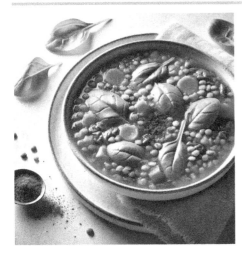

Number of servings: 4
Preparation time: 10 minutes
Cooking time: 30 minutes

Ingredients:

- 1 cup lentils, rinsed
- 6 cups vegetable broth
- 2 cups fresh spinach, chopped
- 2 large carrots, diced
- 1 large onion, diced
- 2 cloves garlic, minced
- 1 tbsp olive oil
- 1 tsp cumin
- 1 tsp paprika
- Salt and pepper to taste

Directions:

1. Heat olive oil in a large pot over medium heat.
2. Add onion and garlic, and sauté until the onion is translucent, about 5 minutes.
3. Stir in carrots, cumin, and paprika, and cook for another 2 minutes.
4. Add lentils and vegetable broth. After bringing to a boil, lower the heat, and cook the lentils until they are soft, about 20 minutes.
5. Stir in chopped spinach and cook for another 5 minutes until wilted.
6. Season with salt and pepper to taste.
7. Serve warm.

Nutritional value per serving:
Calories: 280, Carbs: 40g, Fiber: 15g, Sugars: 7g, Protein: 15g, Saturated fat: 1g, Unsaturated fat: 5g

Difficulty rating: ★★☆☆

Tips for ingredient variations:
Add diced tomatoes or a squeeze of lemon juice for extra flavor.

Chicken Fajitas with Bell Peppers, Onions, and Whole Wheat Tortilla

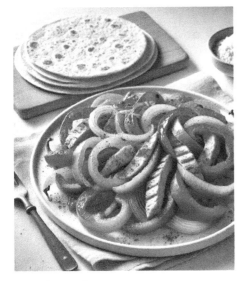

Number of servings: 2
Preparation time: 10 minutes
Cooking time: 15 minutes

Ingredients:

- 2 boneless, skin-free chicken breasts, sliced into strips
- 1 sliced red bell pepper
- 1 sliced green bell pepper
- 1 yellow bell pepper, sliced
- 1 large onion, sliced
- 2 tbsp olive oil
- 1 tsp chili powder
- 1 tsp cumin
- 1 tsp paprika
- 1/2 tsp garlic powder
- Salt and pepper to taste
- 2 whole wheat tortillas

Directions:

1. In a large bowl, mix the chicken strips with chili powder, cumin, paprika, garlic powder, salt, and pepper.
2. In a big skillet, heat the olive oil over medium-high heat.
3. Add chicken strips and cook until browned and cooked through, about 5-7 minutes.
4. Take out the chicken and place it aside from the skillet.
5. In the same skillet, add the bell peppers and onions. Sauté until tender, about 5-7 minutes.
6. Return the chicken to the skillet and mix with the vegetables.
7. Fill whole wheat tortillas with chicken and veggies.

Nutritional value per serving:
Calories: 350, Carbs: 40g, Fiber: 8g, Sugars: 6g, Protein: 28g, Saturated fat: 2g, Unsaturated fat: 10g

Difficulty rating: ★★☆☆

Tips for ingredient variations:
Top with a dollop of Greek yogurt or salsa for added flavor.

Grilled Portobello Mushrooms with Quinoa and Veggies

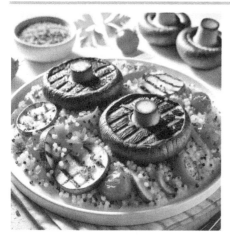

Number of servings: 2

Preparation time: 10 minutes

Cooking time: 20 minutes

Ingredients:

- 4 large portobello mushrooms, stems removed
- 1 cup quinoa, rinsed
- 2 cups vegetable broth
- 1 cup mixed vegetables (zucchini, bell peppers, tomatoes), diced
- 2 tbsp olive oil
- 2 cloves garlic, minced
- 1 tsp balsamic vinegar
- Salt and pepper to taste
- Fresh parsley for garnish

Directions:

1. Cook quinoa in vegetable broth according to package instructions.
2. While the quinoa is cooking, preheat the grill to medium-high heat.
3. Brush the portobello mushrooms with 1 tbsp olive oil and season with salt and pepper.
4. Grill the mushrooms for about 5 minutes on each side, until tender.
5. In a skillet, heat the remaining olive oil over medium heat. For approximately a minute, add the garlic and sauté it until fragrant.
6. Add mixed vegetables to the skillet and cook until tender, about 5-7 minutes.
7. Mix cooked quinoa with the sautéed vegetables and season with balsamic vinegar, salt, and pepper.
8. Serve the grilled portobello mushrooms topped with the quinoa and vegetable mixture. Garnish with fresh parsley.

Nutritional value per serving: Calories: 310, Carbs: 45g, Fiber: 10g, Sugars: 8g, Protein: 10g, Saturated fat: 2g, Unsaturated fat: 10g

Difficulty rating: ★★☆☆☆

Tips for ingredient variations: Add a sprinkle of feta cheese or toasted pine nuts for extra flavor.

Stir-fried Broccoli and Beef with Brown Rice

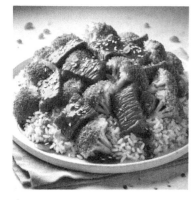

Number of servings: 2

Preparation time: 10 minutes

Cooking time: 20 minutes

Ingredients:

- 8 oz beef sirloin, thinly sliced
- 2 cups broccoli florets
- 1 cup cooked brown rice
- 2 tbsp soy sauce (low sodium)
- 1 tbsp oyster sauce
- 1 tbsp sesame oil
- 1 clove garlic, minced
- 1 tsp ginger, grated
- 1 small onion, sliced
- 1 tbsp cornstarch
- 2 tbsp water
- Salt and pepper to taste

Directions:

1. Combine the oyster sauce, water, and soy sauce in a small bowl. Set aside.
2. In a separate bowl, toss the beef slices with cornstarch until evenly coated.
3. Heat sesame oil in a large skillet or wok over medium-high heat.
4. Add garlic, ginger, and onion, and sauté until fragrant, about 2 minutes.
5. Add the beef to the skillet and cook until browned, about 5 minutes. Remove the beef and set aside.
6. Add the broccoli florets to the same skillet and stir-fry them for 3–4 minutes, or until they are crisp-tender.
7. Return the beef to the skillet and pour in the sauce mixture. Stir well to combine and cook for another 2 minutes.
8. On top of cooked brown rice, serve the stir-fried meat and broccoli.

Nutritional value per serving: Calories: 380, Carbs: 40g, Fiber: 6g, Sugars: 5g, Protein: 30g, Saturated fat: 4g, Unsaturated fat: 12g

Difficulty rating: ★★☆☆☆

Tips for ingredient variations: Add red pepper flakes for a spicy kick or cashews for added crunch.

Cabbage Rolls with Ground Turkey and Brown Rice

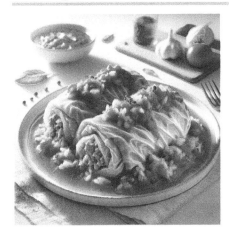

Number of servings: 4
Preparation time: 20 minutes
Cooking time: 60 minutes

Ingredients:

- 8 large cabbage leaves
- 1 lb ground turkey
- 1 cup cooked brown rice
- 1 small onion, finely chopped
- 2 cloves garlic, minced
- 1 tsp dried oregano
- 1 tsp dried thyme
- 1 can (15 oz) tomato sauce
- Salt and pepper to taste

Directions:

1. Preheat the oven to 375°F (190°C).
2. In a large pot, bring water to a boil.Cook the cabbage leaves for two to three minutes, or until they become tender. After draining, set away.
3. In a large bowl, combine the ground turkey, cooked brown rice, onion, garlic, oregano, thyme, salt, and pepper.
4. Lay a cabbage leaf flat and place a portion of the turkey mixture in the center. Enclose the filling by rolling up and folding in the sides. Repeat with the remaining leaves and filling.
5. Place the cabbage rolls seam-side down in a baking dish. Pour the tomato sauce over the rolls.
6. Cover with aluminum foil and bake for 60 minutes, or until the turkey is cooked through.
7. Remove from the oven and let rest for 5 minutes before serving.

Nutritional value per serving:
Calories: 340, Carbs: 25g, Fiber: 5g, Sugars: 8g, Protein: 28g, Saturated fat: 1g, Unsaturated fat: 8g

Difficulty rating: ★★★☆☆

Tips for ingredient variations: Substitute ground turkey with ground chicken or beef for a different flavor.

Baked Chicken Thighs with Brussels Sprouts and Potatoes

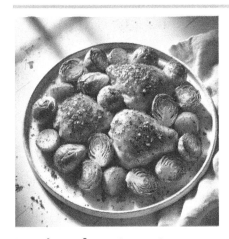

Number of servings: 4
Preparation time: 15 minutes
Cooking time: 40 minutes

Ingredients:

- 4 bone-in, skin-on chicken thighs
- 1 lb Brussels sprouts, halved
- 2 medium potatoes, diced
- 2 tbsp olive oil
- 1 tsp garlic powder
- 1 tsp paprika
- Salt and pepper to taste

Directions:

1. Preheat the oven to 400°F (200°C).
2. In a large bowl, toss the Brussels sprouts and potatoes with 1 tbsp olive oil, garlic powder, paprika, salt, and pepper.
3. Place the chicken thighs on a baking sheet and rub with the remaining olive oil, salt, and pepper.
4. Arrange the Brussels sprouts and potatoes around the chicken on the baking sheet.
5. Bake for 40 minutes, or until the chicken reaches an internal temperature of 165°F (74°C) and the vegetables are tender.
6. Remove from the oven and let rest for 5 minutes before serving.

Nutritional value per serving:
Calories: 350, Carbs: 20g, Fiber: 5g, Sugars: 3g, Protein: 26g, Saturated fat: 5g, Unsaturated fat: 12g

Difficulty rating: ★★☆☆☆

Tips for ingredient variations: Add other root vegetables like carrots or sweet potatoes for additional flavor and nutrients.

Shrimp and Avocado Salad with Lime Dressing

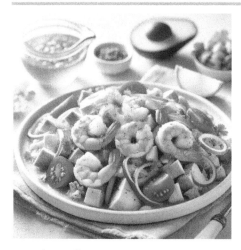

Number of servings: 4
Preparation time: 15 minutes
Cooking time: 5 minutes

Ingredients:

- 1 lb shrimp, peeled and deveined
- 2 avocados, diced
- 1 cup of halved cherry tomatoes
- 1/2 red onion, finely chopped
- 1/4 cup fresh cilantro, chopped
- 2 tbsp olive oil
- Juice of 2 limes
- Salt and pepper to taste

Directions:

1. Heat 1 tbsp of olive oil in a large skillet over medium heat. Add the shrimp and cook for 2-3 minutes on each side until pink and opaque. Remove from heat and let cool.
2. In a large bowl, combine the diced avocado, cherry tomatoes, red onion, and cilantro.
3. In a small bowl, whisk together the remaining olive oil, lime juice, salt, and pepper.
4. Add the cooked shrimp to the salad and drizzle with the lime dressing.
5. Serve right away after gently tossing to mix everything.

Nutritional value per serving: Calories: 300, Carbs: 10g, Fiber: 7g, Sugars: 2g, Protein: 25g, Saturated fat: 2g, Unsaturated fat: 18g

Difficulty rating: ★★☆☆☆

Tips for ingredient variations: Add a dash of hot sauce to the dressing for a spicy kick.

Chicken and Black Bean Burrito Bowl with Brown Rice

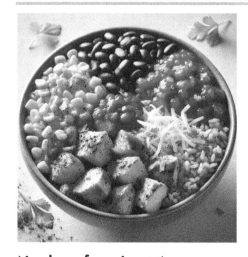

Number of servings: 4
Preparation time: 15 minutes
Cooking time: 30 minutes

Ingredients:

- 1 lb boneless, skinless chicken breasts, diced
- 1 cup cooked brown rice
- 1 can (15 oz) black beans, drained and rinsed
- 1 cup corn kernels
- 1 cup salsa
- 1/2 cup shredded cheddar cheese
- 1/4 cup fresh cilantro, chopped
- 1 tbsp olive oil
- 1 tsp chili powder
- 1 tsp cumin
- Salt and pepper to taste

Directions:

1. Heat the olive oil in a large skillet over medium heat. Add the diced chicken, chili powder, cumin, salt, and pepper. Cook for 8 to 10 minutes, until the chicken is thoroughly cooked and browned.
2. In a large bowl, combine the cooked brown rice, black beans, corn, and salsa.
3. Divide the rice mixture among four bowls.
4. Top each bowl with the cooked chicken, shredded cheese, and fresh cilantro.
5. Serve immediately.

Nutritional value per serving: Calories: 380, Carbs: 45g, Fiber: 10g, Sugars: 5g, Protein: 32g, Saturated fat: 5g, Unsaturated fat: 10g

Difficulty rating: ★★☆☆☆

Tips for ingredient variations: Add diced avocado or a dollop of Greek yogurt for extra creaminess.

Spaghetti Squash with Turkey Bolognese and Parmesan

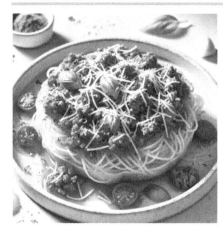

Number of servings: 4
Preparation time: 15 minutes
Cooking time: 40 minutes

Ingredients:

- 1 large spaghetti squash
- 1 lb ground turkey
- 1 can (15 oz) crushed tomatoes
- 1 small onion, finely chopped
- 2 cloves garlic, minced
- 1 tsp dried basil
- 1 tsp dried oregano
- 1/4 cup grated Parmesan cheese
- 1 tbsp olive oil
- Salt and pepper to taste

Directions:

1. Preheat the oven to 400°F (200°C).
2. Cut the spaghetti squash in half lengthwise and remove the seeds. On a baking sheet, place the halves cut-side down. Bake for 30 to 40 minutes, or until soft.
3. In the meantime, place a big skillet over medium heat with the olive oil. Add the onion and garlic, and cook until softened, about 3 minutes.
4. Add the ground turkey, basil, oregano, salt, and pepper. Cook for 8 to 10 minutes, until the turkey is browned and cooked through.
5. Stir in the crushed tomatoes and simmer for 10 minutes.
6. Once the spaghetti squash is done, use a fork to scrape out the strands into a large bowl.
7. Divide the spaghetti squash among four plates and top with the turkey Bolognese sauce.
8. Sprinkle with grated Parmesan cheese and serve.

Nutritional value per serving:
Calories: 330, Carbs: 25g, Fiber: 6g, Sugars: 8g, Protein: 29g, Saturated fat: 3g, Unsaturated fat: 10g

Difficulty rating: ★★☆☆☆

Tips for ingredient variations: Substitute ground turkey with ground chicken or beef for a different flavor.

Grilled Tuna with Mixed Greens and Quinoa

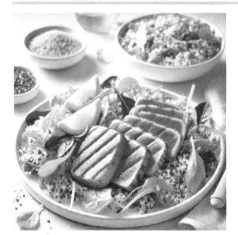

Number of servings: 1
Preparation time: 10 minutes
Cooking time: 10 minutes

Ingredients:

- 4 oz tuna steak
- 1 cup mixed greens
- 1/2 cup cooked quinoa
- 1 tbsp olive oil
- 1 tbsp lemon juice
- Salt and pepper to taste

Directions:

1. Preheat a grill or grill pan over medium-high heat.
2. Sprinkle some salt and pepper on the tuna steak.
3. Grill the tuna for about 3-4 minutes on each side, or until it reaches desired doneness.
4. In a bowl, combine mixed greens and cooked quinoa.
5. Drizzle with olive oil and lemon juice, tossing to coat.
6. Slice the grilled tuna and place it on top of the salad mixture.
7. Serve immediately.

Nutritional value per serving:
Calories: 320, Carbs: 26g, Fiber: 4g, Sugars: 2g, Protein: 30g, Saturated fat: 1g, Unsaturated fat: 10g

Difficulty rating: ★★☆☆☆

Tips for ingredient variations: Add cherry tomatoes or avocado slices for extra flavor and nutrients.

Chicken Caesar Salad (Light Dressing, Whole Wheat Croutons)

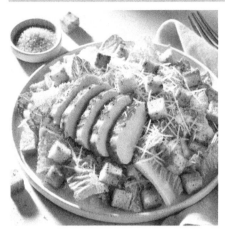

Number of servings: 1
Preparation time: 10 minutes
Cooking time: 15 minutes

Ingredients:

- 4 oz grilled chicken breast, sliced
- 2 cups romaine lettuce, chopped
- 2 tbsp light Caesar dressing
- 1/4 cup whole wheat croutons
- 1 tbsp grated Parmesan cheese

Directions:

1. Combine the light Caesar dressing with the chopped romaine lettuce in a big bowl.
2. Top with sliced grilled chicken breast.
3. Sprinkle with whole wheat croutons and grated Parmesan cheese.
4. Serve immediately.

Nutritional value per serving:
Calories: 300, Carbs: 18g, Fiber: 4g, Sugars: 2g, Protein: 30g, Saturated fat: 3g, Unsaturated fat: 8g

Difficulty rating: ★☆☆☆☆

Tips for ingredient variations: Substitute grilled chicken with grilled shrimp or tofu for a different protein option.

Zucchini Lasagna with Ground Turkey

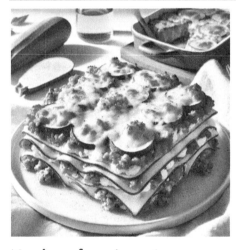

Number of servings: 4
Preparation time: 20 minutes
Cooking time: 40 minutes

Ingredients:

- 3 medium zucchinis, sliced lengthwise into thin strips
- 1 lb ground turkey
- 2 cups marinara sauce
- 1 cup ricotta cheese
- 1 cup shredded mozzarella cheese
- 1/2 cup grated Parmesan cheese
- 1 egg
- 1 tsp dried basil
- 1 tsp dried oregano
- Salt and pepper to taste

Directions:

1. Preheat the oven to 375°F (190°C).
2. In a large skillet, cook the ground turkey over medium heat until browned. Add the marinara sauce and simmer for 10 minutes.
3. In a bowl, mix together the ricotta cheese, egg, dried basil, dried oregano, salt, and pepper.
4. In a baking dish, layer half of the zucchini slices, followed by half of the turkey marinara sauce, and half of the ricotta mixture. Repeat the layers.
5. Top with shredded mozzarella and grated Parmesan cheese.
6. Cover with foil and bake for 30 minutes. Take off the foil and continue baking for ten more minutes, or until the cheese turns golden and bubbling.
7. Before serving, let it cool for a couple of minutes.

Nutritional value per serving:
Calories: 380, Carbs: 16g, Fiber: 4g, Sugars: 7g, Protein: 40g, Saturated fat: 8g, Unsaturated fat: 10g

Difficulty rating: ★★★☆☆

Tips for ingredient variations: Add sliced mushrooms or spinach for extra vegetables.

Vegetable and Bean Tacos with Whole Wheat Tortilla

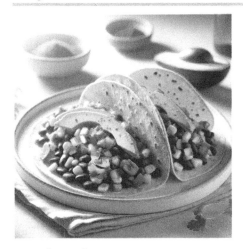

Number of servings: 2

Preparation time: 10 minutes

Cooking time: 10 minutes

Ingredients:

- 4 whole wheat tortillas
- 1 cup black beans, drained and rinsed
- 1 cup corn kernels
- 1 red bell pepper, diced
- 1/2 red onion, diced
- 1 avocado, sliced
- 1/4 cup cilantro, chopped
- 1 tbsp olive oil
- 1 tsp ground cumin
- 1 tsp chili powder
- Salt and pepper to taste

Directions:

1. Heat the olive oil in a pan over medium heat.
2. Saute the diced red onion and bell pepper for approximately five minutes, until they become tender.
3. Stir in the black beans, corn, ground cumin, chili powder, salt, and pepper. Cook for an additional 5 minutes.
4. Warm the whole wheat tortillas in a separate skillet or microwave.
5. Divide the vegetable and bean mixture among the tortillas.
6. Top with sliced avocado and chopped cilantro.
7. Serve immediately.

Nutritional value per serving: Calories: 320, Carbs: 44g, Fiber: 12g, Sugars: 4g, Protein: 10g, Saturated fat: 2g, Unsaturated fat: 10g

Difficulty rating: ★☆☆☆☆

Tips for ingredient variations: Add a squeeze of lime juice or a dollop of Greek yogurt for extra flavor.

Turkey and Spinach Stuffed Mushrooms with Cheese

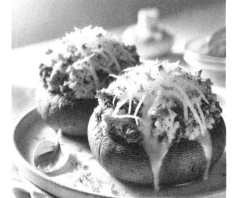

Number of servings: 2

Preparation time: 15 minutes

Cooking time: 20 minutes

Ingredients:

- 8 large portobello mushrooms, stems removed
- 1/2 lb ground turkey
- 1 cup fresh spinach, chopped
- 1/2 cup ricotta cheese
- 1/2 cup shredded mozzarella cheese
- 1/4 cup grated Parmesan cheese
- 1 egg
- 1 tsp dried basil
- 1 tsp dried oregano
- Salt and pepper to taste
- 1 tbsp olive oil

Directions:

1. Preheat the oven to 375°F (190°C).
2. Heat the olive oil in a pan over medium heat. Add the ground turkey and cook until browned.
3. Add the chopped spinach and heat, stirring, until it wilts. Take off the heat and allow to cool a little.
4. In a bowl, mix together the ricotta cheese, shredded mozzarella, grated Parmesan, egg, dried basil, dried oregano, salt, and pepper.
5. Stir in the cooked turkey and spinach mixture.
6. Place the mushroom caps on a baking sheet and fill each with the turkey mixture.
7. Bake for 20 minutes, or until the mushrooms are tender and the filling is golden.
8. Serve immediately.

Nutritional value per serving: Calories: 300, Carbs: 10g, Fiber: 3g, Sugars: 4g, Protein: 38g, Saturated fat: 8g, Unsaturated fat: 10g

Difficulty rating: ★★★☆☆

Tips for ingredient variations: Substitute turkey with ground chicken or beef for a different flavor profile.

Grilled Chicken with Cauliflower Mash and Green Beans

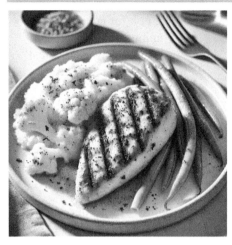

Number of servings: 1
Preparation time: 10 minutes
Cooking time: 20 minutes

Ingredients:

- 1 chicken breast (4 oz)
- 1 cup cauliflower florets
- 1 tbsp unsalted butter
- 1/4 cup low-fat milk
- 1 cup green beans, trimmed
- 1 tbsp olive oil
- Salt and pepper to taste
- 1 tsp garlic powder

Directions:

1. Preheat the grill to medium-high heat.
2. Add salt, pepper, and garlic powder to the chicken breast to season. Grill for about 6-8 minutes per side, or until fully cooked and juices run clear.
3. Meanwhile, steam the cauliflower florets until tender, about 10 minutes. Drain and transfer to a blender or food processor. Add the butter and milk, then blend until smooth. Season with salt and pepper to taste.
4. Heat the olive oil in a pan over medium heat. Add the green beans and simmer for about 5 minutes, until they are crisp-tender. Season with salt and pepper.
5. Serve the grilled chicken alongside the cauliflower mash and green beans.

Nutritional value per serving: Calories: 320, Carbs: 12g, Fiber: 5g, Sugars: 4g, Protein: 38g, Saturated fat: 6g, Unsaturated fat: 8g

Difficulty rating: ★★☆☆☆

Tips for ingredient variations: Add a squeeze of lemon juice over the chicken for extra flavor.

Fish Tacos with Cabbage Slaw and Salsa

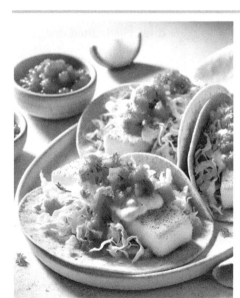

Number of servings: 2
Preparation time: 15 minutes
Cooking time: 10 minutes

Ingredients:

- 8 oz white fish fillets (e.g., tilapia or cod)
- 4 small whole wheat tortillas
- 1 cup shredded cabbage
- 1/4 cup Greek yogurt
- 1 tbsp lime juice
- 1/2 cup salsa
- 1 tbsp olive oil
- Salt and pepper to taste
- 1 tsp chili powder
- 1/2 tsp cumin

Directions:

1. Preheat the oven to 400°F (200°C).
2. Add cumin, chili powder, salt, and pepper to the fish fillets' seasoning. Arrange on a baking tray and brush with olive oil. Fish should flake readily with a fork after 10 minutes of baking.
3. In a bowl, mix the shredded cabbage with Greek yogurt and lime juice. Season with salt and pepper to taste.
4. Warm the tortillas in the oven for 1-2 minutes or in a skillet over medium heat.
5. Assemble the tacos by placing a piece of fish on each tortilla, topping with cabbage slaw and salsa.
6. Serve immediately.

Nutritional value per serving: Calories: 380, Carbs: 40g, Fiber: 10g, Sugars: 4g, Protein: 30g, Saturated fat: 4g, Unsaturated fat: 8g

Difficulty rating: ★★☆☆☆

Tips for ingredient variations: Add sliced avocado or pickled onions for extra flavor and texture.

Baked Eggplant Parmesan with Marinara Sauce

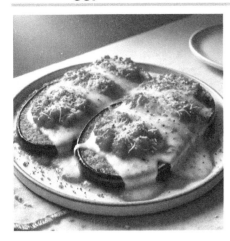

Number of servings: 2
Preparation time: 15 minutes
Cooking time: 30 minutes

Ingredients:

- 1 large eggplant, sliced into 1/2-inch rounds
- 1 cup marinara sauce
- 1/2 cup shredded mozzarella cheese (low-fat)
- 1/4 cup grated Parmesan cheese
- 1/2 cup whole wheat breadcrumbs
- 1 egg, beaten
- 1 tbsp olive oil
- Salt and pepper to taste
- 1 tsp dried basil

Directions:

1. Preheat the oven to 375°F (190°C). Line a baking sheet with parchment paper.
2. To extract moisture, salt the eggplant slices and leave them for ten minutes. Pat dry with a paper towel.
3. Dip each eggplant slice in the beaten egg, then coat with breadcrumbs.
4. Arrange the eggplant slices on the baking sheet and drizzle with olive oil. Bake until golden brown, turning once during the 20 minutes of baking.
5. Spread a thin layer of marinara sauce in a baking dish. Arrange the baked eggplant slices in the dish, top with remaining marinara sauce, and sprinkle with mozzarella and Parmesan cheese.
6. Bake for an additional 10 minutes, until the cheese is melted and bubbly.
7. Sprinkle with dried basil before serving.

Nutritional value per serving: Calories: 340, Carbs: 40g, Fiber: 12g, Sugars: 14g, Protein: 15g, Saturated fat: 4g, Unsaturated fat: 8g

Difficulty rating: ★★☆☆☆

Tips for ingredient variations: Use fresh basil leaves for a more aromatic flavor.

Beef and Vegetable Kebabs with Quinoa

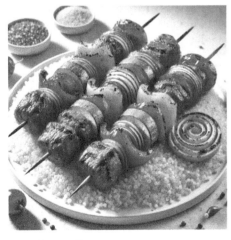

Number of servings: 2
Preparation time: 20 minutes
Cooking time: 15 minutes

Ingredients:

- 8 oz beef sirloin, cut into 1-inch cubes
- 1 red bell pepper, cut into 1-inch pieces
- 1 yellow bell pepper, cut into 1-inch pieces
- 1 red onion, cut into wedges
- 1 zucchini, sliced into 1/2-inch rounds
- 1 cup cooked quinoa
- 1 tbsp olive oil
- 1 tbsp soy sauce
- 1 tbsp lemon juice
- 1 tsp garlic powder
- Salt and pepper to taste

Directions:

1. Preheat the grill to medium-high heat.
2. In a bowl, mix olive oil, soy sauce, lemon juice, garlic powder, salt, and pepper. Add beef cubes and marinate for 15 minutes.
3. Thread beef and vegetables onto skewers, alternating pieces.
4. Grill kebabs for 10-15 minutes, turning occasionally, until beef is cooked to desired doneness.
5. Serve kebabs over a bed of cooked quinoa.

Nutritional value per serving: Calories: 350, Carbs: 30g, Fiber: 6g, Sugars: 6g, Protein: 30g, Saturated fat: 4g, Unsaturated fat: 12g

Difficulty rating: ★★☆☆☆

Tips for ingredient variations: Add cherry tomatoes or mushrooms to the kebabs for additional flavor.

Chicken and Mango Salad with Mixed Greens

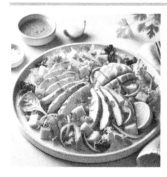

Number of servings: 2

Preparation time: 10 minutes

Ingredients:

- 2 cups mixed greens
- 1 cooked chicken breast, sliced
- 1 ripe mango, diced
- 1/4 cup red onion, thinly sliced
- 1/4 cup chopped cilantro
- 1 tbsp olive oil
- 1 tbsp lime juice
- Salt and pepper to taste

Directions:

1. In a large bowl, combine mixed greens, sliced chicken, diced mango, red onion, and cilantro.
2. Mix the olive oil, lime juice, salt, and pepper in a small bowl.
3. Over the salad, drizzle with the dressing and toss lightly to mix.
4. Serve immediately.

Nutritional value per serving: Calories: 300, Carbs: 22g, Fiber: 5g, Sugars: 17g, Protein: 26g, Saturated fat: 2g, Unsaturated fat: 8g

Difficulty rating: ★☆☆☆☆

Tips for ingredient variations: Add avocado slices or cherry tomatoes for extra flavor and nutrients.

Quinoa and Black Bean Stuffed Peppers with Salsa

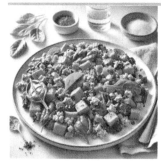

Number of servings: 2

Preparation time: 15 minutes

Cooking time: 30 minutes

Ingredients:

- 2 large bell peppers, halved and seeded
- 1 cup cooked quinoa
- 1 cup black beans, rinsed and drained
- 1/2 cup corn kernels
- 1/2 cup diced tomatoes
- 1/4 cup chopped cilantro
- 1 tsp cumin
- 1 tsp chili powder
- Salt and pepper to taste
- 1/2 cup salsa

Directions:

1. Preheat the oven to 375°F (190°C).
2. In a large bowl, combine the cooked quinoa, black beans, corn, diced tomatoes, cilantro, cumin, chili powder, salt, and pepper.
3. Fill the bell pepper halves with the mixture of quinoa.Serve right away.
4. Cover the filled peppers with foil after placing them in a roasting dish.
5. Bake for 30 minutes, or until the peppers are tender.
6. Serve with salsa on top.

Nutritional value per serving: Calories: 340, Carbs: 60g, Fiber: 15g, Sugars: 9g, Protein: 12g, Saturated fat: 1g, Unsaturated fat: 2g

Difficulty rating: ★★☆☆☆

Tips for ingredient variations: Add shredded cheese on top before baking for a richer flavor.

Turkey and Sweet Potato Hash with Spinach

Number of servings: 2

Preparation time: 10 minutes

Cooking time: 20 minutes

Ingredients:

- 1 large sweet potato, peeled and diced
- 1/2 lb ground turkey
- 1 cup fresh spinach, chopped
- 1 small onion, diced
- 1 red bell pepper, diced
- 1 tbsp olive oil
- Salt and pepper to taste
- 1/2 tsp paprika

Directions:

1. Heat the olive oil in a large skillet over medium heat.
2. Add the diced sweet potato and cook for about 10 minutes, stirring occasionally, until tender.
3. Add the onion and red bell pepper, cooking for an additional 5 minutes.
4. Add the ground turkey to the skillet after pushing the veggies to one side. Cook until browned and cooked through, breaking it up with a spoon.
5. Stir in the spinach and cook until wilted.
6. Season with salt, pepper, and paprika.
7. Serve hot.

Nutritional value per serving: Calories: 380, Carbs: 35g, Fiber: 7g, Sugars: 8g, Protein: 28g, Saturated fat: 3g, Unsaturated fat: 7g

Difficulty rating: ★★☆☆☆

Tips for ingredient variations: Substitute ground turkey with ground chicken or beef if desired.

Grilled Salmon with Quinoa and Asparagus

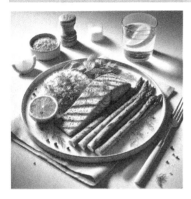

Number of servings: 2
Preparation time: 10 minutes
Cooking time: 20 minutes

Ingredients:

- 2 salmon fillets (about 4 oz each)
- 1 cup cooked quinoa
- 1 bunch asparagus, trimmed
- 1 tbsp olive oil
- 1 lemon, sliced
- Salt and pepper to taste
- 1 tsp dried dill

Directions:

1. Preheat the grill to medium-high heat.
2. In addition to seasoning with salt, pepper, and dill, drizzle the salmon fillets and asparagus with olive oil.
3. Cook the salmon on the grill for 4–5 minutes on each side, or until it reaches the desired doneness.
4. When the asparagus is tender, grill it for five to seven minutes, flipping it occasionally.
5. Serve the salmon with quinoa and grilled asparagus, garnished with lemon slices.

Nutritional value per serving: Calories: 380, Carbs: 25g, Fiber: 5g, Sugars: 3g, Protein: 34g, Saturated fat: 2g, Unsaturated fat: 10g

Difficulty rating: ★★☆☆

Tips for ingredient variations: Add a sprinkle of parmesan cheese to the asparagus for extra flavor.

Chicken and Avocado Salad with Mixed Greens

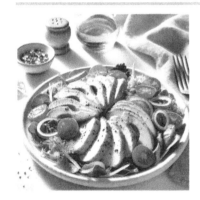

Number of servings: 2
Preparation time: 10 minutes

Ingredients:

- 2 cups mixed greens
- 1 cooked chicken breast, sliced
- 1 avocado, diced
- 1/2 cup cherry tomatoes, halved
- 1/4 cup red onion, thinly sliced
- 2 tbsp olive oil
- 1 tbsp balsamic vinegar
- Salt and pepper to taste

Directions:

1. In a large salad bowl, combine the mixed greens, sliced chicken, avocado, cherry tomatoes, and red onion.
2. In a small bowl, whisk together the olive oil, balsamic vinegar, salt, and pepper.
3. Over the salad, drizzle with the dressing and toss lightly to mix.
4. Serve immediately.

Nutritional value per serving: Calories: 310, Carbs: 12g, Fiber: 7g, Sugars: 3g, Protein: 25g, Saturated fat: 3g, Unsaturated fat: 17g

Difficulty rating: ★☆☆☆

Tips for ingredient variations: Add crumbled feta cheese or toasted nuts for extra texture and flavor.

Vegetable Stuffed Bell Peppers with Quinoa

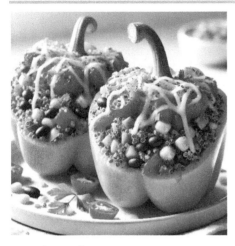

Number of servings: 2
Preparation time: 15 minutes
Cooking time: 30 minutes

Ingredients:

- 2 large bell peppers, halved and seeded
- 1 cup cooked quinoa
- 1/2 cup black beans, rinsed and drained
- 1/2 cup corn kernels
- 1/2 cup diced tomatoes
- 1/4 cup chopped cilantro
- 1 tsp cumin
- 1 tsp chili powder
- Salt and pepper to taste
- 1/2 cup shredded cheddar cheese

Directions:

1. Preheat the oven to 375°F (190°C).
2. In a large bowl, combine the cooked quinoa, black beans, corn, diced tomatoes, cilantro, cumin, chili powder, salt, and pepper.
3. Fill the bell pepper halves with the mixture of quinoa.Serve right away.
4. Place the stuffed peppers in a baking dish and sprinkle the shredded cheddar cheese on top.
5. Cover with foil and bake for 30 minutes, or until the peppers are tender and the cheese is melted.
6. Serve hot.

Nutritional value per serving: Calories: 340, Carbs: 54g, Fiber: 12g, Sugars: 8g, Protein: 14g, Saturated fat: 4g, Unsaturated fat: 4g

Difficulty rating: ★★☆☆☆

Tips for ingredient variations: Substitute cheddar cheese with mozzarella or add some cooked ground turkey for additional protein.

Tuna Salad Lettuce Wraps with Avocado

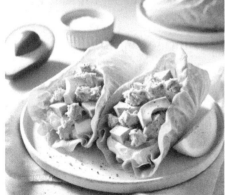

Number of servings: 1
Preparation time: 10 minutes

Ingredients:

- 1 can (5 oz) tuna in water, drained
- 1/4 avocado, diced
- 1 tbsp Greek yogurt (low-fat)
- 1 tbsp lemon juice
- 1 tbsp red onion, finely chopped
- Salt and pepper to taste
- 4 large lettuce leaves

Directions:

1. In a bowl, combine the tuna, avocado, Greek yogurt, lemon juice, and red onion.
2. Mix well and season with salt and pepper to taste.
3. Spoon the tuna salad mixture onto the center of each lettuce leaf.
4. Roll up the lettuce leaves to create wraps.
5. Serve immediately.

Nutritional value per serving: Calories: 290, Carbs: 7g, Fiber: 4g, Sugars: 1g, Protein: 33g, Saturated fat: 1g, Unsaturated fat: 11g

Difficulty rating: ★☆☆☆☆

Tips for ingredient variations: Add diced cucumber or bell pepper for extra crunch and flavor.

Chickpea and Spinach Stew with Brown Rice

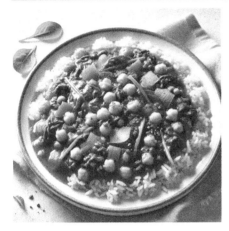

Number of servings: 2
Preparation time: 10 minutes
Cooking time: 25 minutes

Ingredients:

- 1 cup chickpeas, cooked
- 2 cups fresh spinach, chopped
- 1/2 cup brown rice, uncooked
- 1 small onion, chopped
- 2 cloves garlic, minced
- 1 tbsp olive oil
- 1 cup vegetable broth
- 1 tsp cumin
- 1 tsp paprika
- Salt and pepper to taste

Directions:

1. Cook the brown rice according to package instructions.
2. Heat the olive oil in a big pot over medium heat.
3. Add the chopped onion and garlic, and sauté until translucent, about 5 minutes.
4. Add the cumin and paprika, and cook for another minute.
5. Stir in the chickpeas and vegetable broth, and bring to a simmer.
6. Cook the chopped spinach for three to four minutes, until it wilts.
7. Season with salt and pepper to taste.
8. Serve the stew over a bed of brown rice.

Nutritional value per serving: Calories: 310, Carbs: 47g, Fiber: 8g, Sugars: 3g, Protein: 10g, Saturated fat: 1g, Unsaturated fat: 6g

Difficulty rating: ★★☆☆

Tips for ingredient variations: Add diced tomatoes or carrots for extra texture and flavor.

Turkey and Zucchini Skewers with Couscous

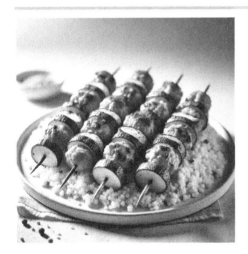

Number of servings: 2
Preparation time: 15 minutes
Cooking time: 15 minutes

Ingredients:

- 1 lb ground turkey
- 1 medium zucchini, sliced
- 1/4 cup breadcrumbs
- 1 egg
- 2 cloves garlic, minced
- 1 tbsp fresh parsley, chopped
- Salt and pepper to taste
- 1 cup couscous, cooked
- 1 tbsp olive oil

Directions:

1. In a bowl, combine the ground turkey, breadcrumbs, egg, garlic, parsley, salt, and pepper. Mix well.
2. Form the mixture into small meatballs and thread onto skewers alternately with zucchini slices.
3. Heat the olive oil in a grill pan over medium heat.
4. Cook the skewers, turning occasionally, until the turkey is cooked through and the zucchini is tender, about 12-15 minutes.
5. Place the kebabs on top of the cooked couscous.

Nutritional value per serving: Calories: 340, Carbs: 34g, Fiber: 4g, Sugars: 2g, Protein: 29g, Saturated fat: 3g, Unsaturated fat: 7g

Difficulty rating: ★★☆☆

Tips for ingredient variations: Add cherry tomatoes or bell peppers to the skewers for extra flavor and color.

Lemon Garlic Shrimp with Asparagus and Quinoa

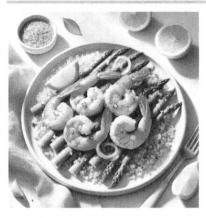

Number of servings: 2
Preparation time: 10 minutes
Cooking time: 20 minutes

Ingredients:

- 1 lb shrimp, peeled and deveined
- 1 bunch asparagus, trimmed and cut into pieces
- 1 cup quinoa, cooked
- 2 cloves garlic, minced
- 2 tbsp lemon juice
- 1 tbsp olive oil
- Salt and pepper to taste
- Fresh parsley, chopped (optional)

Directions:

1. Cook the quinoa according to package instructions.
2. In a large skillet, heat the olive oil over medium heat.
3. Add the garlic and cook for one minute, until fragrant.
4. Add the shrimp and asparagus, and cook until the shrimp is pink and opaque, and the asparagus is tender, about 5-7 minutes.
5. Add the lemon juice and season to taste with salt and pepper.
6. Serve the shrimp and asparagus over a bed of quinoa, and garnish with fresh parsley if desired.

Nutritional value per serving: Calories: 330, Carbs: 31g, Fiber: 5g, Sugars: 2g, Protein: 32g, Saturated fat: 1g, Unsaturated fat: 7g

Difficulty rating: ★★☆☆

Tips for ingredient variations: Add a pinch of red pepper flakes for a bit of heat.

Chicken and Vegetable Kebabs with Brown Rice

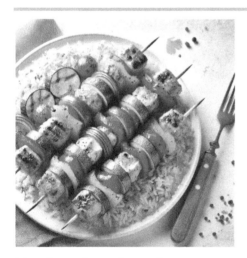

Number of servings: 2
Preparation time: 20 minutes
Cooking time: 20 minutes

Ingredients:

- 1 lb chicken breast, cut into cubes
- 1 red bell pepper, cut into pieces
- 1 yellow bell pepper, cut into pieces
- 1 zucchini, sliced
- 1 red onion, cut into pieces
- 1 cup brown rice, cooked
- 2 tbsp olive oil
- 2 tbsp lemon juice
- 2 cloves garlic, minced
- Salt and pepper to taste
- Fresh herbs (parsley, cilantro) for garnish

Directions:

1. In a bowl, combine the olive oil, lemon juice, garlic, salt, and pepper. Add the chicken cubes and marinate for at least 15 minutes.
2. Preheat the grill to medium-high heat.
3. Thread the chicken, bell peppers, zucchini, and onion onto skewers.
4. Grill the kebabs, turning occasionally, until the chicken is cooked through and the vegetables are tender, about 15-20 minutes.
5. Serve the kebabs over a bed of cooked brown rice and garnish with fresh herbs.

Nutritional value per serving: Calories: 350, Carbs: 35g, Fiber: 5g, Sugars: 6g, Protein: 30g, Saturated fat: 2g, Unsaturated fat: 10g

Difficulty rating: ★★☆☆

Tips for ingredient variations: Add mushrooms or cherry tomatoes to the skewers for added flavor and nutrition.

SIDE DISHES

Steamed Broccoli with Lemon Zest

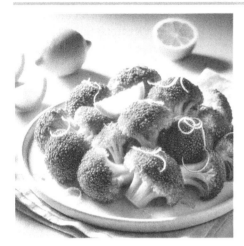

Number of servings: 2
Preparation time: 5 minutes
Cooking time: 5 minutes

Ingredients:

- 2 cups broccoli florets
- 1 tbsp lemon zest
- Salt to taste

Directions:

1. Fill a pot with water and bring it to a boil. Put a steamer basket over the pot.
2. After placing the broccoli florets in the steamer basket, cover it. Steam the broccoli for approximately five minutes, or until it is soft.
3. Remove the broccoli from the steamer and place in a serving bowl.
4. Sprinkle lemon zest over the broccoli and season with salt to taste.
5. Serve warm.

Nutritional value per serving: Calories: 25, Carbs: 5g, Fiber: 2g, Sugars: 2g, Protein: 2g, Saturated fat: 0g, Unsaturated fat: 0g

Difficulty rating: ★☆☆☆☆

Tips for ingredient variations: Add a dash of freshly ground black pepper or a drizzle of olive oil for added flavor.

Roasted Brussels Sprouts with Balsamic Glaze

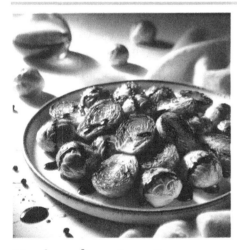

Number of servings: 2
Preparation time: 10 minutes
Cooking time: 20 minutes

Ingredients:

- 2 cups Brussels sprouts, halved
- 1 tbsp olive oil
- 1 tbsp balsamic vinegar
- Salt and pepper to taste

Directions:

1. Preheat the oven to 400°F (200°C).
2. Toss the halved Brussels sprouts with olive oil, salt, and pepper.
3. Spread the Brussels sprouts on a baking sheet in a single layer.
4. Roast in the preheated oven for about 20 minutes, or until tender and slightly caramelized.
5. Drizzle the balsamic vinegar over the roasted Brussels sprouts and toss to coat.
6. Serve immediately.

Nutritional value per serving: Calories: 35, Carbs: 7g, Fiber: 3g, Sugars: 3g, Protein: 2g, Saturated fat: 0g, Unsaturated fat: 2g

Difficulty rating: ★★☆☆☆

Tips for ingredient variations: Add a sprinkle of grated Parmesan cheese before serving for a savory twist.

Garlic Green Beans with Almonds

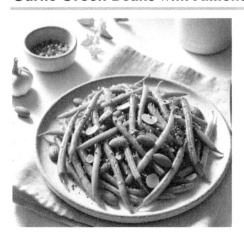

Number of servings: 2
Preparation time: 5 minutes
Cooking time: 10 minutes

Ingredients:

- 2 cups green beans, trimmed
- 1 tbsp olive oil
- 2 cloves garlic, minced
- 2 tbsp sliced almonds
- Salt and pepper to taste

Directions:

1. Heat olive oil in a large skillet over medium heat.
2. Add the minced garlic and simmer for one minute, or until fragrant.
3. Add the green beans and cook, stirring frequently, until tender, about 5-7 minutes.
4. Add the sliced almonds and cook for an additional 2 minutes, stirring frequently.
5. Season with salt and pepper to taste.
6. Serve warm.

Nutritional value per serving: Calories: 30, Carbs: 5g, Fiber: 2g, Sugars: 2g, Protein: 1g, Saturated fat: 0g, Unsaturated fat: 2g

Difficulty rating: ★★☆☆☆

Tips for ingredient variations: Substitute almonds with chopped walnuts or pecans for a different nutty flavor.

Cucumber and Tomato Salad with Feta

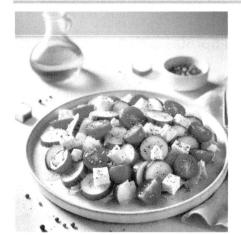

Number of servings: 2
Preparation time: 10 minutes

Ingredients:

- 1 cup cucumber, diced
- 1 cup of halved cherry tomatoes
- 1/4 cup feta cheese, crumbled
- 1 tbsp olive oil
- 1 tbsp lemon juice
- Salt and pepper to taste

Directions:

1. In a large bowl, combine the diced cucumber and halved cherry tomatoes.
2. Drizzle with olive oil and lemon juice.
3. Add the crumbled feta cheese and toss to combine.
4. Season with salt and pepper to taste.
5. Serve immediately.

Nutritional value per serving: Calories: 30, Carbs: 3g, Fiber: 1g, Sugars: 2g, Protein: 1g, Saturated fat: 1g, Unsaturated fat: 2g

Difficulty rating: ★☆☆☆☆

Tips for ingredient variations: Add fresh herbs like basil or mint for additional flavor.

Sauteed Spinach with Garlic and Olive Oil

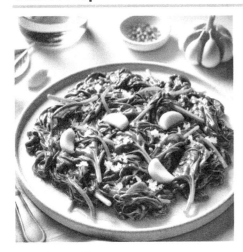

Number of servings: 2
Preparation time: 5 minutes
Cooking time: 5 minutes

Ingredients:

- 4 cups fresh spinach
- 1 tbsp olive oil
- 2 cloves garlic, minced
- Salt and pepper to taste

Directions:

1. Heat the olive oil in a large skillet over medium heat.
2. Add the minced garlic and simmer for one minute, or until fragrant.
3. Add the fresh spinach and cook, stirring frequently, until wilted, about 2-3 minutes.
4. Season with salt and pepper to taste.
5. Serve warm.

Nutritional value per serving:
Calories: 30, Carbs: 4g, Fiber: 2g, Sugars: 0g, Protein: 1g, Saturated fat: 0g, Unsaturated fat: 2g

Difficulty rating: ★☆☆☆☆

Tips for ingredient variations:
Add a splash of lemon juice or a pinch of red pepper flakes for added zest.

Cauliflower Rice with Herbs

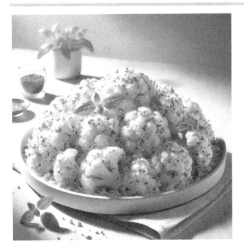

Number of servings: 2
Preparation time: 10 minutes
Cooking time: 5 minutes

Ingredients:

- 1 medium cauliflower, riced (about 4 cups)
- 1 tbsp olive oil
- 1 tsp dried parsley
- 1 tsp dried basil
- Salt and pepper to taste

Directions:

1. Heat the olive oil in a large skillet over medium heat.
2. Add the riced cauliflower to the skillet and cook for about 5 minutes, stirring occasionally, until the cauliflower is tender.
3. Stir in the dried parsley and basil.
4. Season with salt and pepper to taste.
5. Serve warm.

Nutritional value per serving:
Calories: 40, Carbs: 5g, Fiber: 2g, Sugars: 2g, Protein: 2g, Saturated fat: 0g, Unsaturated fat: 2g

Difficulty rating: ★☆☆☆☆

Tips for ingredient variations:
Add a squeeze of lemon juice for a fresh, tangy flavor.

Grilled Asparagus with Parmesan

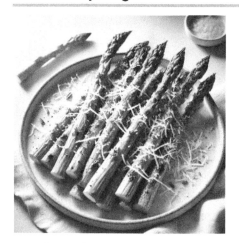

Number of servings: 2
Preparation time: 5 minutes
Cooking time: 10 minutes

Ingredients:

- 1 bunch asparagus, trimmed
- 1 tbsp olive oil
- 2 tbsp grated Parmesan cheese
- Salt and pepper to taste

Directions:

1. Preheat the grill to medium-high heat.
2. Toss the asparagus with olive oil, salt, and pepper.
3. Grill the asparagus for about 8-10 minutes, turning occasionally, until tender and slightly charred.
4. Sprinkle the grilled asparagus with grated Parmesan cheese.
5. Serve immediately.

Nutritional value per serving: Calories: 60, Carbs: 4g, Fiber: 2g, Sugars: 2g, Protein: 4g, Saturated fat: 1g, Unsaturated fat: 3g

Difficulty rating: ★☆☆☆☆

Tips for ingredient variations: Add a pinch of garlic powder or red pepper flakes for extra flavor.

Zucchini Noodles with Pesto

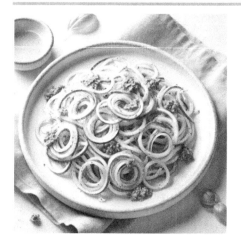

Number of servings: 2
Preparation time: 10 minutes
Cooking time: 5 minutes

Ingredients:

- 2 medium zucchinis, spiralized
- 2 tbsp pesto sauce (store-bought or homemade)
- 1 tbsp olive oil
- Salt and pepper to taste

Directions:

1. Heat the olive oil in a large skillet over medium heat.
2. Add the spiralized zucchini noodles to the skillet and cook for about 3-5 minutes, until tender.
3. Take off the heat source and combine the pesto sauce with the zucchini noodles.
4. Season with salt and pepper to taste.
5. Serve warm.

Nutritional value per serving: Calories: 40, Carbs: 3g, Fiber: 1g, Sugars: 2g, Protein: 1g, Saturated fat: 0g, Unsaturated fat: 3g

Difficulty rating: ★☆☆☆☆

Tips for ingredient variations: Top with cherry tomatoes or a sprinkle of Parmesan cheese for added flavor and texture.

Baked Sweet Potato Fries with Paprika

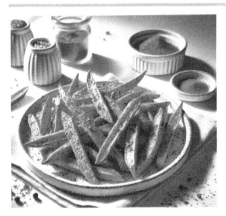

Number of servings: 2
Preparation time: 10 minutes
Cooking time: 25 minutes

Ingredients:

- 2 medium sweet potatoes, cut into fries
- 1 tbsp olive oil
- 1 tsp paprika
- Salt and pepper to taste

Directions:

1. Preheat the oven to 425°F (220°C).
2. Toss the sweet potato fries with olive oil, paprika, salt, and pepper.
3. Spread the fries in a single layer on a baking sheet.
4. Bake for 20-25 minutes, turning halfway through, until crispy and golden brown.
5. Serve immediately.

Nutritional value per serving: Calories: 100, Carbs: 20g, Fiber: 3g, Sugars: 7g, Protein: 2g, Saturated fat: 1g, Unsaturated fat: 4g

Difficulty rating: ★☆☆☆☆

Tips for ingredient variations: Add a sprinkle of garlic powder or cayenne pepper for extra flavor.

Mixed Greens with Balsamic Vinaigrette and Walnuts

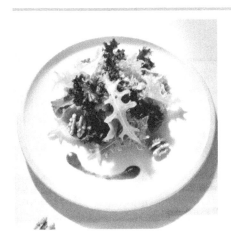

Number of servings: 2
Preparation time: 5 minutes

Ingredients:

- 4 cups mixed greens
- 1/4 cup walnuts, chopped
- 2 tbsp balsamic vinaigrette

Directions:

1. In a large bowl, toss the mixed greens with balsamic vinaigrette.
2. Top with chopped walnuts.
3. Serve immediately.

Nutritional value per serving: Calories: 70, Carbs: 4g, Fiber: 2g, Sugars: 2g, Protein: 2g, Saturated fat: 0g, Unsaturated fat: 5g

Difficulty rating: ★☆☆☆☆

Tips for ingredient variations: Add sliced strawberries or crumbled feta cheese for additional flavor and texture.

Roasted Carrots with Thyme and Honey

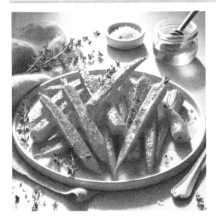

Number of servings: 4
Preparation time: 10 minutes
Cooking time: 25 minutes

Ingredients:

- 1 lb carrots, peeled and cut into sticks
- 2 tbsp olive oil
- 1 tbsp honey
- 1 tsp dried thyme
- Salt and pepper to taste

Directions:

1. Preheat the oven to 400°F (200°C).
2. In a large bowl, toss the carrot sticks with olive oil, honey, thyme, salt, and pepper.
3. Spread the carrots in a single layer on a baking sheet.
4. Roast in the preheated oven for 25 minutes, or until tender and slightly caramelized.
5. Serve warm.

Nutritional value per serving: Calories: 80, Carbs: 13g, Fiber: 3g, Sugars: 8g, Protein: 1g, Saturated fat: 1g, Unsaturated fat: 6g

Difficulty rating: ★☆☆☆☆

Tips for ingredient variations: Add a squeeze of fresh lemon juice after roasting for a tangy flavor.

Kale Chips with Nutritional Yeast

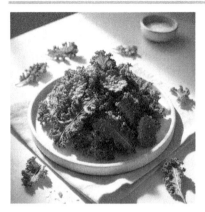

Number of servings: 2
Preparation time: 10 minutes
Cooking time: 15 minutes

Ingredients:

- 1 bunch of cleaned and shredded kale into small pieces
- 1 tbsp olive oil
- 2 tbsp nutritional yeast
- Salt to taste

Directions:

1. Preheat the oven to 350°F (175°C).
2. In a large bowl, toss the kale pieces with olive oil, nutritional yeast, and salt.
3. Spread the kale in a single layer on a baking sheet.
4. Bake for 15 minutes, or until the edges are crispy but not burnt.
5. Serve immediately.

Nutritional value per serving:
Calories: 70, Carbs: 5g, Fiber: 2g, Sugars: 1g, Protein: 3g, Saturated fat: 1g, Unsaturated fat: 5g

Difficulty rating: ★☆☆☆☆

Tips for ingredient variations:
Add a pinch of smoked paprika or garlic powder for additional flavor.

Tomato Basil Salad with Mozzarella

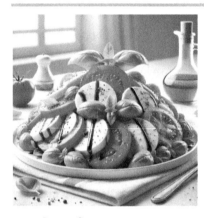

Number of servings: 4
Preparation time: 10 minutes

Ingredients:

- 4 medium tomatoes, sliced
- 1/2 cup fresh basil leaves
- 4 oz fresh mozzarella, sliced
- 2 tbsp balsamic vinegar
- 1 tbsp olive oil
- Salt and pepper to taste

Directions:

1. Arrange the tomato slices on a serving platter.
2. Top with fresh basil leaves and mozzarella slices.
3. Drizzle with balsamic vinegar and olive oil.
4. Season with salt and pepper to taste.
5. Serve immediately.

Nutritional value per serving:
Calories: 50, Carbs: 4g, Fiber: 1g, Sugars: 3g, Protein: 3g, Saturated fat: 1g, Unsaturated fat: 3g

Difficulty rating: ★☆☆☆☆

Tips for ingredient variations:
Add a few slices of avocado or a sprinkle of pine nuts for added texture and flavor.

Mashed Cauliflower with Garlic

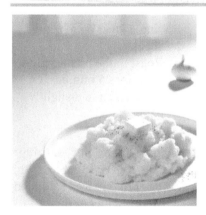

Number of servings: 4
Preparation time: 10 minutes
Cooking time: 15 minutes

Ingredients:

- 1 large head cauliflower, cut into florets
- 2 cloves garlic, minced
- 2 tbsp butter
- 1/4 cup low-fat milk
- Salt and pepper to taste

Directions:

1. Bring a large pot of water to a boil. Add the cauliflower florets and cook until tender, about 10 minutes.
2. Drain the cauliflower and transfer to a blender or food processor.
3. Add the minced garlic, butter, and milk. Blend until smooth and creamy.
4. Season with salt and pepper to taste.
5. Serve warm.

Nutritional value per serving:
Calories: 70, Carbs: 7g, Fiber: 3g, Sugars: 3g, Protein: 3g, Saturated fat: 2g, Unsaturated fat: 2g

Difficulty rating: ★☆☆☆☆

Tips for ingredient variations:
Add a sprinkle of grated Parmesan cheese for extra flavor.

Quinoa Pilaf with Vegetables

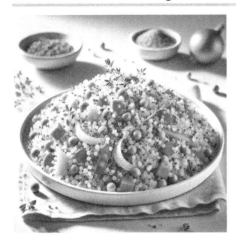

Number of servings: 4
Preparation time: 10 minutes
Cooking time: 20 minutes

Ingredients:

- 1 cup quinoa, rinsed
- 2 cups low-sodium vegetable broth
- 1 tbsp olive oil
- 1 small onion, diced
- 1 bell pepper, diced
- 1 carrot, diced
- 1/2 cup peas
- 1 tsp dried thyme
- Salt and pepper to taste

Directions:

1. In a medium pot, heat the olive oil over medium heat. Add the onion, bell pepper, and carrot, and sauté until tender, about 5 minutes.
2. Add the quinoa and vegetable broth to the pot. Bring to a boil.
3. After 15 minutes, or until the quinoa is cooked and the liquid has been absorbed, reduce the heat to low, cover, and simmer.
4. Stir in the peas and thyme. Season with salt and pepper to taste.
5. Serve warm.

Nutritional value per serving:
Calories: 90, Carbs: 16g, Fiber: 3g, Sugars: 3g, Protein: 3g, Saturated fat: 1g, Unsaturated fat: 3g

Difficulty rating: ★☆☆☆

Tips for ingredient variations:
Add a handful of chopped fresh herbs like parsley or cilantro for added freshness.

Roasted Butternut Squash with Cinnamon

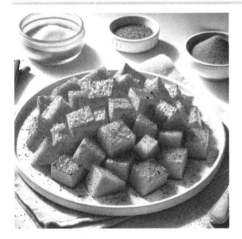

Number of servings: 4
Preparation time: 10 minutes
Cooking time: 30 minutes

Ingredients:

- 1 medium butternut squash, peeled and cubed
- 2 tbsp olive oil
- 1 tsp ground cinnamon
- 1/2 tsp salt
- 1/4 tsp black pepper

Directions:

1. Preheat the oven to 400°F (200°C).
2. In a large bowl, toss the butternut squash cubes with olive oil, ground cinnamon, salt, and black pepper until evenly coated.
3. Spread the squash cubes in a single layer on a baking sheet lined with parchment paper.
4. Roast the squash for 25 to 30 minutes in a preheated oven, stirring halfway through, or until it is soft and golden brown.
5. Serve warm.

Nutritional value per serving:
Calories: 100, Carbs: 16g, Fiber: 3g, Sugars: 3g, Protein: 1g, Saturated fat: 1g, Unsaturated fat: 5g

Difficulty rating: ★☆☆☆

Tips for ingredient variations:
Add a pinch of nutmeg or allspice for extra flavor.

Carrot and Ginger Soup with Coconut Milk

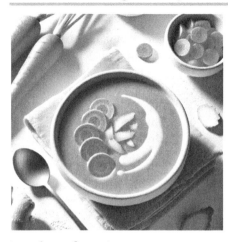

Number of servings: 4
Preparation time: 10 minutes
Cooking time: 20 minutes

Ingredients:

- 1 lb carrots, peeled and chopped
- 1 small onion, chopped
- 2 cloves garlic, minced
- 1 tbsp ginger, grated
- 1 tbsp olive oil
- 3 cups vegetable broth
- 1 cup light coconut milk
- Salt and pepper to taste

Directions:

1. Heat the olive oil in a big pot over medium heat.
2. Add the chopped onion, garlic, and grated ginger. Cook until the onion is soft, about 5 minutes.
3. Add the chopped carrots and vegetable broth. Bring to a boil, then reduce the heat and simmer until the carrots are tender, about 15 minutes.
4. Use an immersion blender to puree the soup until smooth, or transfer to a blender in batches.
5. Stir in the coconut milk and season with salt and pepper to taste. Heat through before serving.

Nutritional value per serving: Calories: 80, Carbs: 10g, Fiber: 2g, Sugars: 4g, Protein: 1g, Saturated fat: 2g, Unsaturated fat: 2g

Difficulty rating: ★★☆☆☆

Tips for ingredient variations: Garnish with fresh cilantro or a squeeze of lime juice for added freshness.

Sauteed Mushrooms with Thyme

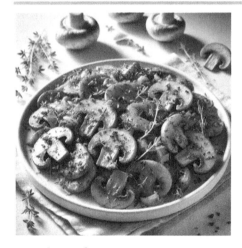

Number of servings: 4
Preparation time: 5 minutes
Cooking time: 10 minutes

Ingredients:

- 1 lb mushrooms, sliced
- 2 tbsp olive oil
- 1 tbsp fresh thyme leaves
- 2 cloves garlic, minced
- Salt and pepper to taste

Directions:

1. Heat the olive oil in a large skillet over medium-high heat.
2. Add the sliced mushrooms and simmer for approximately 5 minutes, stirring now and again, until the juices come out and they begin to brown.
3. Add the minced garlic and fresh thyme leaves. Cook for another 2-3 minutes, until the garlic is fragrant and the mushrooms are tender.
4. Season with salt and pepper to taste and serve warm.

Nutritional value per serving: Calories: 60, Carbs: 5g, Fiber: 2g, Sugars: 2g, Protein: 2g, Saturated fat: 1g, Unsaturated fat: 4g

Difficulty rating: ★☆☆☆☆

Tips for ingredient variations: Add a splash of balsamic vinegar for a tangy twist.

Steamed Snap Peas with Sesame Seeds

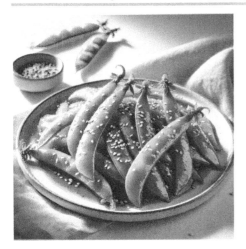

Number of servings: 4
Preparation time: 5 minutes

Cooking time: 5 minutes

Ingredients:

- 1 lb snap peas, trimmed
- 1 tbsp sesame seeds, toasted
- 1 tbsp soy sauce
- 1 tsp sesame oil

Directions:

1. Steam the snap peas in a steamer basket over boiling water until tender-crisp, about 3-5 minutes.
2. Transfer the snap peas to a serving bowl.
3. Drizzle with soy sauce and sesame oil.
4. Sprinkle with toasted sesame seeds and toss to coat evenly.
5. Serve warm.

Nutritional value per serving:
Calories: 50, Carbs: 7g, Fiber: 2g, Sugars: 3g, Protein: 3g, Saturated fat: 0g, Unsaturated fat: 2g

Difficulty rating: ★☆☆☆☆

Tips for ingredient variations: Add a pinch of red pepper flakes for a spicy kick.

Roasted Beet Salad with Goat Cheese

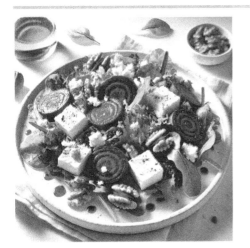

Number of servings: 4
Preparation time: 10 minutes
Cooking time: 40 minutes

Difficulty rating: ★★☆☆☆

Ingredients:

- 4 medium beets, washed and trimmed
- 2 tbsp olive oil
- 2 oz goat cheese, crumbled
- 2 cups mixed greens
- 1/4 cup walnuts, toasted
- 1 tbsp balsamic vinegar
- Salt and pepper to taste

Directions:

1. Preheat the oven to 400°F (200°C).
2. Wrap each beet in aluminum foil and place on a baking sheet. Roast in the preheated oven for 35-40 minutes, or until tender when pierced with a fork.
3. Allow the beets to cool, then peel and cut into cubes.
4. In a large bowl, combine the mixed greens, roasted beets, crumbled goat cheese, and toasted walnuts.
5. Drizzle with olive oil and balsamic vinegar. Toss to coat evenly.
6. Season with salt and pepper to taste and serve.

Nutritional value per serving:
Calories: 90, Carbs: 10g, Fiber: 3g, Sugars: 7g, Protein: 3g, Saturated fat: 2g, Unsaturated fat: 6g

Tips for ingredient variations: Add sliced avocado or orange segments for extra flavor and nutrients.

SNACKS

Apple Slices with Almond Butter and Raisins

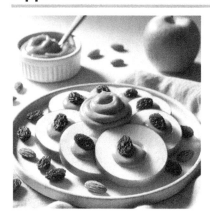

Number of servings: 1
Preparation time: 5 minutes

Ingredients:

- 1 medium apple, sliced
- 1 tbsp almond butter
- 1 tbsp raisins

Directions:

1. Core and slice the apple into thin wedges.
2. Spread the almond butter evenly over the apple slices.
3. Sprinkle raisins over the almond butter-topped apple slices.
4. Serve immediately.

Nutritional value per serving: Calories: 150, Carbs: 27g, Fiber: 5g, Sugars: 20g, Protein: 2g, Saturated fat: 0g, Unsaturated fat: 6g

Difficulty rating: ★☆☆☆☆

Tips for ingredient variations: Use peanut butter or cashew butter instead of almond butter for a different flavor.

Carrot Sticks with Hummus and Paprika

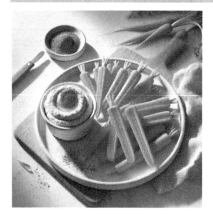

Number of servings: 1
Preparation time: 5 minutes

Ingredients:

- 1 cup carrot sticks
- 2 tbsp hummus
- 1/4 tsp paprika

Directions:

1. Arrange the carrot sticks on a serving plate.
2. Place the hummus in a small bowl.
3. Sprinkle paprika over the hummus.
4. Enjoy the carrot sticks dipped in hummus.

Nutritional value per serving: Calories: 120, Carbs: 19g, Fiber: 5g, Sugars: 8g, Protein: 3g, Saturated fat: 0g, Unsaturated fat: 3g

Difficulty rating: ★☆☆☆☆

Tips for ingredient variations: Substitute paprika with cumin or chili powder for a different spice.

Greek Yogurt with Honey and Walnuts 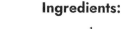 Almonds

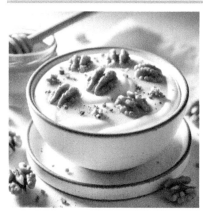

Number of servings: 1
Preparation time: 5 minutes

Ingredients:

- 1/2 cup Greek yogurt (low-fat)
- 1 tsp honey
- 1 tbsp chopped walnuts

Directions:

1. Transfer the Greek yogurt into a bowl.
2. Pour honey over the yogurt.
3. Sprinkle chopped walnuts on top.
4. Stir gently to combine all ingredients and serve immediately.

Nutritional value per serving: Calories: 140, Carbs: 14g, Fiber: 1g, Sugars: 12g, Protein: 10g, Saturated fat: 1g, Unsaturated fat: 4g

Difficulty rating: ★☆☆☆☆

Tips for ingredient variations: Add a pinch of cinnamon or a few fresh berries for extra flavor.

The Dr. Now 1200-Calorie Diet Plan

Mixed Nuts (1 oz) and Dried Fruit

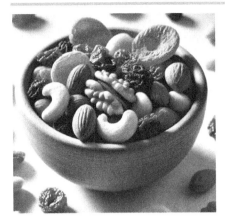

Number of servings: 1
Preparation time: 5 minutes

Ingredients:

- 1 oz mixed nuts (almonds, cashews, walnuts)
- 2 tbsp dried fruit (raisins, cranberries, apricots)

Directions:

1. In a small bowl, combine the mixed nuts and dried fruit.
2. Mix well and serve immediately or store in an airtight container for later.

Nutritional value per serving: Calories: 180, Carbs: 20g, Fiber: 3g, Sugars: 12g, Protein: 4g, Saturated fat: 2g, Unsaturated fat: 12g

Difficulty rating: ★☆☆☆☆

Tips for ingredient variations: Use your favorite combination of nuts and dried fruits to customize this snack.

Celery Sticks with Peanut Butter and Raisins

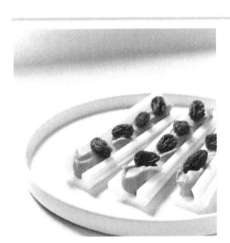

Number of servings: 1
Preparation time: 5 minutes

Ingredients:

- 2 large celery sticks
- 1 tbsp peanut butter
- 1 tbsp raisins

Directions:

1. Cut the celery sticks into smaller pieces if desired.
2. Spread peanut butter into the hollow part of each celery stick.
3. Over the peanut butter, scatter the raisins.
4. Serve immediately.

Nutritional value per serving: Calories: 150, Carbs: 16g, Fiber: 3g, Sugars: 10g, Protein: 4g, Saturated fat: 1g, Unsaturated fat: 7g

Difficulty rating: ★☆☆☆☆

Tips for ingredient variations: Try almond butter or sunflower seed butter for a different taste.

Sliced Bell Peppers with Guacamole and Lime

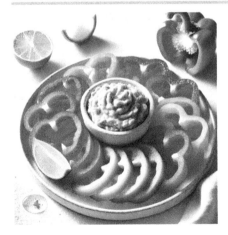

Number of servings: 1
Preparation time: 10 minutes

Ingredients:

- 1 large bell pepper, sliced
- 1/4 cup guacamole
- 1/2 lime, juiced

Directions:

1. Wash and slice the bell pepper into strips.
2. Place the guacamole in a small serving dish.
3. Squeeze the lime juice over the bell pepper slices.
4. Serve the bell pepper slices with guacamole for dipping.

Nutritional value per serving: Calories: 130, Carbs: 16g, Fiber: 7g, Sugars: 5g, Protein: 2g, Saturated fat: 1g, Unsaturated fat: 8g

Difficulty rating: ★☆☆☆☆

Tips for ingredient variations: Add a sprinkle of paprika or cayenne pepper to the guacamole for a spicy kick.

Cottage Cheese with Pineapple and Chia Seeds

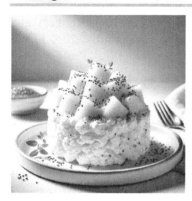

Number of servings: 1
Preparation time: 5 minutes

Ingredients:

- 1/2 cup low-fat cottage cheese
- 1/4 cup pineapple chunks (fresh or canned in juice, drained)
- 1 tsp chia seeds

Directions:

1. In a bowl, combine the cottage cheese and pineapple chunks.
2. Sprinkle chia seeds on top.
3. Stir gently to mix all ingredients together.
4. Serve immediately.

Nutritional value per serving: Calories: 120, Carbs: 12g, Fiber: 3g, Sugars: 8g, Protein: 10g, Saturated fat: 1g, Unsaturated fat: 2g

Difficulty rating: ★☆☆☆☆

Tips for ingredient variations: Use fresh berries or diced mango instead of pineapple for a different flavor.

Cherry Tomatoes and Mozzarella Balls with Basil

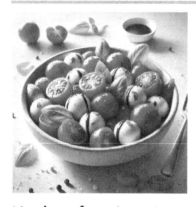

Number of servings: 1
Preparation time: 10 minutes

Ingredients:

- 1 cup of halved cherry tomatoes
- 1/4 cup small mozzarella balls (bocconcini)
- 1 tbsp fresh basil, chopped
- 1 tsp balsamic vinegar
- Salt and pepper to taste

Directions:

1. In a bowl, combine the cherry tomatoes and mozzarella balls.
2. Add the chopped basil and gently toss to mix.
3. Drizzle with balsamic vinegar and season with salt and pepper to taste.
4. Serve immediately.

Nutritional value per serving: Calories: 140, Carbs: 7g, Fiber: 2g, Sugars: 5g, Protein: 9g, Saturated fat: 3g, Unsaturated fat: 4g

Difficulty rating: ★☆☆☆☆

Tips for ingredient variations: Add a few olives or a sprinkle of oregano for an extra burst of flavor.

Protein Bar with Dark Chocolate

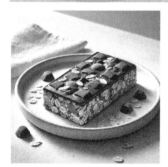

Number of servings: 1
Preparation time: 10 minutes
Ingredients:

- 1/2 cup rolled oats
- 1/4 cup protein powder (vanilla or chocolate flavor)
- 2 tbsp almond butter
- 1 tbsp honey
- 1/4 cup dark chocolate chips (70% cocoa or higher)
- 1/4 cup almond milk (unsweetened)
- 1 tsp vanilla extract

Directions:

1. In a bowl, mix together the rolled oats and protein powder.
2. Add almond butter, honey, dark chocolate chips, almond milk, and vanilla extract. Mix until well combined.
3. Press the mixture into a small baking dish lined with parchment paper.
4. Refrigerate for at least 1 hour until firm.
5. Cut into bars and serve.

Nutritional value per serving: Calories: 200, Carbs: 20g, Fiber: 5g, Sugars: 8g, Protein: 12g, Saturated fat: 4g, Unsaturated fat: 7g

Difficulty rating: ★★☆☆☆

Tips for ingredient variations: Add dried fruit or nuts for additional flavor and texture.

Hard-Boiled Egg with Avocado

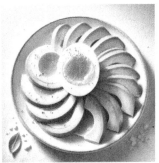

Number of servings: 1

Preparation time: 10 minutes

Ingredients:

- 1 large egg
- 1/4 medium avocado
- Salt and pepper to taste

Directions:

1. Put the egg in a pot and add water to cover it. Bring to a boil over medium-high heat.
2. Once boiling, cover the saucepan and remove from heat. Let the egg sit in the hot water for 9-12 minutes, depending on your preferred level of doneness.
3. Remove the egg from hot water and let it cool under cold running water. Peel the egg.
4. Slice the avocado and place it on a plate.
5. Slice the hard-boiled egg and arrange it alongside the avocado.
6. Season with salt and pepper to taste and serve.

Nutritional value per serving: Calories: 100, Carbs: 6g, Fiber: 4g, Sugars: 1g, Protein: 6g, Saturated fat: 1g, Unsaturated fat: 6g

Difficulty rating: ★☆☆☆☆

Tips for ingredient variations: Add a squeeze of lemon juice over the avocado for extra flavor.

Blueberry Almond Smoothie with Protein Powder

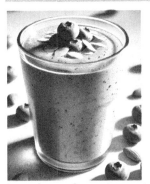

Number of servings: 1

Preparation time: 5 minutes

Ingredients:

- 1/2 cup blueberries
- 1/2 cup unsweetened almond milk
- 1 scoop vanilla protein powder
- 1 tbsp almond butter
- 1/2 cup ice cubes

Directions:

1. Place all ingredients (blueberries, almond milk, protein powder, almond butter, and ice cubes) in a blender.
2. Blend until smooth and creamy.
3. Pour into a glass and serve immediately.

Nutritional value per serving: Calories: 160, Carbs: 12g, Fiber: 4g, Sugars: 6g, Protein: 15g, Saturated fat: 0.5g, Unsaturated fat: 6g

Difficulty rating: ★☆☆☆☆

Tips for ingredient variations: Add a handful of spinach for extra nutrients without altering the taste significantly.

Edamame (1 cup) with Sea Salt

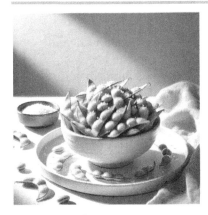

Number of servings: 1

Preparation time: 5 minutes

Cooking time: 5 minutes

Ingredients:

- 1 cup edamame (in pods or shelled)
- 1/4 tsp sea salt

Directions:

1. Bring a pot of water to a boil.
2. Add the edamame and simmer until soft, about 3 to 5 minutes.
3. Drain the edamame and transfer to a serving bowl.
4. Sprinkle with sea salt and toss to coat evenly.
5. Serve warm or at room temperature.

Nutritional value per serving: Calories: 140, Carbs: 10g, Fiber: 6g, Sugars: 2g, Protein: 12g, Saturated fat: 0.5g, Unsaturated fat: 4g

Difficulty rating: ★☆☆☆☆

Tips for ingredient variations: Add a sprinkle of chili flakes or a dash of soy sauce for a different flavor profile.

Rice Cakes with Avocado and Smoked Salmon

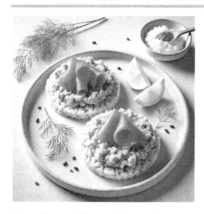

Number of servings: 1
Preparation time: 5 minutes

Ingredients:

- 2 plain rice cakes
- 1/4 medium avocado
- 2 slices smoked salmon
- Fresh dill for garnish (optional)
- Lemon juice (optional)

Directions:

1. Spread the mashed avocado evenly over the two rice cakes.
2. Top each rice cake with a slice of smoked salmon.
3. Garnish with fresh dill and a squeeze of lemon juice, if desired.
4. Serve immediately.

Nutritional value per serving:
Calories: 140, Carbs: 14g, Fiber: 4g, Sugars: 1g, Protein: 8g, Saturated fat: 1g, Unsaturated fat: 6g

Difficulty rating: ★☆☆☆☆

Tips for ingredient variations:
Add a slice of cucumber on top for added crunch and freshness.

Strawberries and Dark Chocolate with Almonds

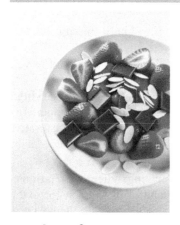

Number of servings: 1
Preparation time: 5 minutes

Ingredients:

- 1/2 cup fresh strawberries, sliced
- 1/2 oz dark chocolate (70% cocoa or higher), chopped
- 1 tbsp almonds, chopped

Directions:

1. Arrange the sliced strawberries on a plate.
2. Sprinkle the chopped dark chocolate over the strawberries.
3. Scatter the chopped almonds on top.
4. Serve immediately and enjoy.

Nutritional value per serving:
Calories: 150, Carbs: 14g, Fiber: 4g, Sugars: 9g, Protein: 3g, Saturated fat: 3g, Unsaturated fat: 6g

Difficulty rating: ★☆☆☆☆

Tips for ingredient variations:
Substitute almonds with walnuts or pecans for a different nutty flavor.

Cucumber Slices with Feta and Olive Oil

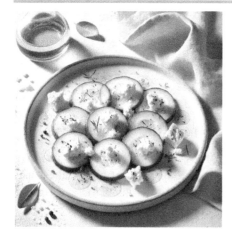

Number of servings: 1
Preparation time: 5 minutes

Ingredients:

- 1 cucumber, sliced
- 1 oz feta cheese, crumbled
- 1 tsp olive oil
- Salt and pepper to taste

Directions:

1. Arrange the cucumber slices on a plate.
2. Sprinkle the crumbled feta cheese evenly over the cucumber slices.
3. Drizzle the olive oil over the top.
4. Season with salt and pepper to taste.
5. Serve immediately.

Nutritional value per serving:
Calories: 120, Carbs: 6g, Fiber: 1g, Sugars: 3g, Protein: 4g, Saturated fat: 2g, Unsaturated fat: 4g

Difficulty rating: ★☆☆☆☆

Tips for ingredient variations:
Add a sprinkle of fresh herbs such as dill or mint for added flavor.

Pumpkin Seeds (1 oz) with Dried Cranberries

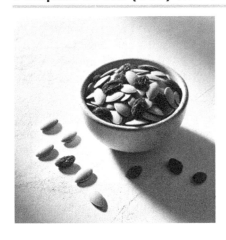

Number of servings: 1
Preparation time: 2 minutes

Ingredients:

- 1 oz pumpkin seeds
- 1 tbsp dried cranberries

Directions:

1. Combine the pumpkin seeds and dried cranberries in a small bowl.
2. Mix well to ensure an even distribution.
3. Serve as a snack.

Nutritional value per serving:
Calories: 150, Carbs: 15g, Fiber: 3g, Sugars: 6g, Protein: 5g, Saturated fat: 1g, Unsaturated fat: 10g

Difficulty rating: ★☆☆☆☆

Tips for ingredient variations:
Add a sprinkle of cinnamon or a dash of sea salt for extra flavor.

Apple and Walnut Salad with Cinnamon

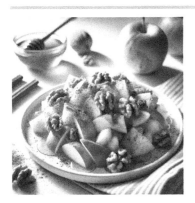

Ingredients:

- 1 apple, cored and diced
- 1/4 cup walnuts, chopped
- 1 tsp ground cinnamon
- 1 tsp honey (optional)

Directions:

1. In a bowl, combine the diced apple and chopped walnuts.
2. Sprinkle with ground cinnamon.
3. Drizzle honey over the top if using.
4. Mix well to coat the apple pieces evenly.
5. Serve immediately.

Number of servings: 1
Preparation time: 5 minutes

Nutritional value per serving:
Calories: 170, Carbs: 22g, Fiber: 5g, Sugars: 15g, Protein: 3g, Saturated fat: 1g, Unsaturated fat: 10g

Difficulty rating: ★☆☆☆☆

Tips for ingredient variations:
Use different types of apples such as Granny Smith or Honeycrisp for varying flavors.

Veggie Sticks with Salsa and Greek Yogurt

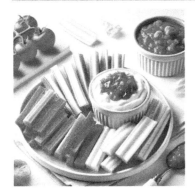

Ingredients:

- 1 carrot, cut into sticks
- 1 celery stalk, cut into sticks
- 1/2 bell pepper, cut into sticks
- 2 tbsp salsa
- 2 tbsp Greek yogurt (low-fat)

Directions:

1. Arrange the veggie sticks on a plate.
2. In a small bowl, mix the salsa and Greek yogurt until well combined.
3. Serve the veggie sticks with the salsa and Greek yogurt dip.

Number of servings: 1
Preparation time: 5 minutes

Nutritional value per serving:
Calories: 100, Carbs: 14g, Fiber: 4g, Sugars: 7g, Protein: 5g, Saturated fat: 1g, Unsaturated fat: 1g

Difficulty rating: ★☆☆☆☆

Tips for ingredient variations:
Use different vegetables such as cucumber, cherry tomatoes, or zucchini sticks for variety.

Protein Shake with Almond Milk

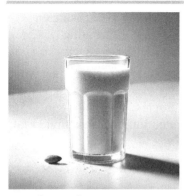

Number of servings: 1

Preparation time: 5 minutes

Ingredients:

- 1 scoop protein powder (choose your preferred flavor)
- 1 cup almond milk (unsweetened)
- 1/2 banana
- 1 tsp honey (optional)
- Ice cubes (optional)

Directions:

1. In a blender, combine the protein powder, almond milk, banana, and honey if using.
2. If you want your shake cold, add some ice cubes.
3. Blend until smooth.
4. Pour into a glass and serve immediately.

Nutritional value per serving: Calories: 200, Carbs: 22g, Fiber: 3g, Sugars: 12g, Protein: 20g, Saturated fat: 1g, Unsaturated fat: 2g

Difficulty rating: ★☆☆☆☆

Tips for ingredient variations: Add a handful of spinach or a tablespoon of nut butter for extra nutrients and flavor.

DESSERTS

Frozen Yogurt Bark with Berries and Nuts

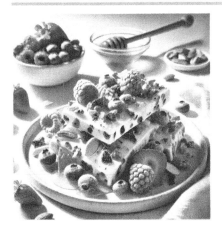

Number of servings: 4
Preparation time: 10 minutes
Freezing time: 2 hours

Ingredients:

- 2 cups Greek yogurt (low-fat)
- 1/2 cup of mixed berries (strawberries, raspberries, and blueberries)
- 1/4 cup chopped nuts (almonds, walnuts, or pistachios)
- 1 tbsp honey

Directions:

1. Line a baking sheet with parchment paper.
2. Spread the Greek yogurt evenly over the parchment paper to about 1/4 inch thickness.
3. Scatter the mixed berries and chopped nuts evenly over the yogurt.
4. Drizzle honey over the top.
5. Place the baking sheet in the freezer and freeze for at least 2 hours, or until firm.
6. Once frozen, break the yogurt bark into pieces.
7. Store in an airtight container in the freezer until ready to eat.

Nutritional value per serving: Calories: 120, Carbs: 15g, Fiber: 2g, Sugars: 11g, Protein: 6g, Saturated fat: 1g, Unsaturated fat: 3g

Difficulty rating: ★☆☆☆☆

Tips for ingredient variations: Substitute honey with maple syrup or agave nectar. Use your favorite nuts or seeds.

Chocolate Avocado Pudding with Berries

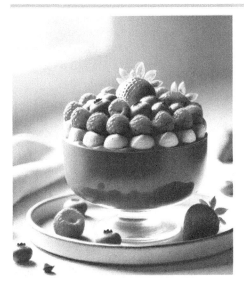

Number of servings: 2
Preparation time: 10 minutes

Ingredients:

- 1 ripe avocado
- 1/4 cup unsweetened cocoa powder
- 1/4 cup almond milk (unsweetened)
- 2 tbsp honey or maple syrup
- 1/2 tsp vanilla extract
- 1/2 cup of mixed berries (strawberries, raspberries, and blueberries)

Directions:

1. In a blender or food processor, combine the avocado, cocoa powder, almond milk, honey or maple syrup, and vanilla extract.
2. Blend until smooth and creamy.
3. Divide the pudding into two bowls.
4. Top with mixed berries.
5. Serve immediately or refrigerate for up to 24 hours.

Nutritional value per serving: Calories: 150, Carbs: 24g, Fiber: 7g, Sugars: 13g, Protein: 3g, Saturated fat: 2g, Unsaturated fat: 10g

Difficulty rating: ★☆☆☆☆

Tips for ingredient variations: Add a pinch of sea salt to enhance the chocolate flavor. Substitute berries with sliced bananas or mango.

Baked Apples with Cinnamon and Walnuts

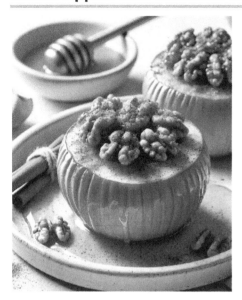

Number of servings: 2
Preparation time: 10 minutes

Cooking time: 20 minutes

Ingredients:

- 2 medium apples
- 2 tsp cinnamon
- 2 tbsp chopped walnuts
- 2 tsp honey

Directions:

1. Preheat the oven to 350°F (175°C).
2. Core the apples and place them in a baking dish.
3. Sprinkle cinnamon evenly inside and on top of the apples.
4. Fill the center of each apple with chopped walnuts.
5. Drizzle honey over the top.
6. Bake in the preheated oven for about 20 minutes, or until the apples are tender.
7. Serve warm.

Nutritional value per serving: Calories: 120, Carbs: 26g, Fiber: 5g, Sugars: 20g, Protein: 1g, Saturated fat: 0g, Unsaturated fat: 3g

Difficulty rating: ★☆☆☆

Tips for ingredient variations: Substitute walnuts with pecans or almonds. Add a dollop of Greek yogurt on top for extra creaminess.

Chia Seed Pudding with Mango and Coconut Milk

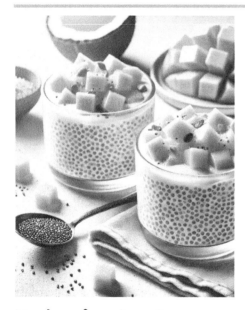

Number of servings: 2
Preparation time: 10 minutes

Chilling time: 2 hours

Ingredients:

- 1/4 cup chia seeds
- 1 cup coconut milk (unsweetened)
- 1 tbsp honey or maple syrup
- 1/2 tsp vanilla extract
- 1 cup diced mango

Directions:

1. Mix the chia seeds, coconut milk, vanilla essence, honey, or maple syrup in a medium-sized bowl.
2. Cover and refrigerate for at least 2 hours, or until the mixture has thickened.
3. To break up any clumps, stir the pudding.
4. Spoon the pudding into two bowls, then sprinkle the diced mango over top.
5. Serve chilled.

Nutritional value per serving: Calories: 140, Carbs: 23g, Fiber: 7g, Sugars: 14g, Protein: 3g, Saturated fat: 4g, Unsaturated fat: 2g

Difficulty rating: ★☆☆☆

Tips for ingredient variations: Substitute mango with your favorite fruit such as strawberries, blueberries, or pineapple.

Greek Yogurt with Honey, Walnuts, and Blueberries

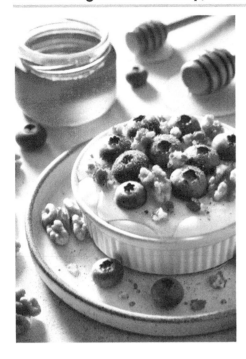

Number of servings: 1

Preparation time: 5 minutes

Ingredients:

- 1 cup Greek yogurt (low-fat)
- 1/4 cup blueberries
- 1 tbsp honey
- 1 tbsp chopped walnuts

Directions:

1. In a bowl, add the Greek yogurt.
2. Top with blueberries.
3. Drizzle honey over the yogurt and berries.
4. Sprinkle chopped walnuts on top.
5. Serve immediately.

Nutritional value per serving: Calories: 150, Carbs: 25g, Fiber: 3g, Sugars: 20g, Protein: 12g, Saturated fat: 1g, Unsaturated fat: 3g

Difficulty rating: ★☆☆☆☆

Tips for ingredient variations: Substitute honey with agave nectar or maple syrup. Use your favorite nuts or seeds for a different crunch.

Fruit Salad with Mint and Lime

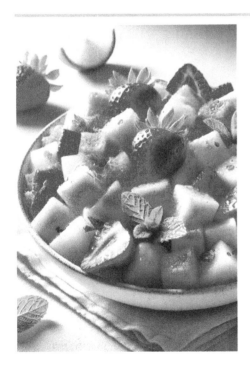

Number of servings: 1

Preparation time: 10 minutes

Ingredients:

- 1/2 cup diced pineapple
- 1/2 cup diced mango
- 1/2 cup diced watermelon
- 1/2 cup halved strawberries
- 1 tbsp fresh mint leaves, chopped
- Juice of 1 lime

Directions:

1. In a large bowl, combine the pineapple, mango, watermelon, and strawberries.
2. Add the chopped mint leaves.
3. Squeeze the lime juice over the fruit and gently toss to combine.
4. Serve right away or store in the fridge until you're ready to eat.

Nutritional value per serving: Calories: 90, Carbs: 23g, Fiber: 3g, Sugars: 19g, Protein: 1g, Saturated fat: 0g, Unsaturated fat: 0g

Difficulty rating: ★☆☆☆☆

Tips for ingredient variations: Add a sprinkle of chia seeds or a drizzle of honey for extra flavor and nutrients.

Banana Ice Cream with Dark Chocolate

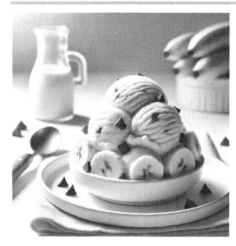

Number of servings: 1
Preparation time: 10 minutes
Freezing time: 2 hours

Ingredients:

- 1 ripe banana
- 1 tbsp dark chocolate chips

Directions:

1. Peel and slice the banana into small pieces.
2. Place the banana slices in a freezer-safe container and freeze for at least 2 hours, or until completely frozen.
3. Once frozen, place the banana slices in a blender or food processor and blend until smooth and creamy.
4. Stir in the dark chocolate chips.
5. Serve immediately as a soft-serve or freeze for an additional 30 minutes for a firmer texture.

Nutritional value per serving:
Calories: 130, Carbs: 31g, Fiber: 3g, Sugars: 18g, Protein: 2g, Saturated fat: 2g, Unsaturated fat: 2g

Difficulty rating: ★☆☆☆☆

Tips for ingredient variations:
Add a splash of vanilla extract or a pinch of cinnamon for additional flavor.

Almond Flour Brownies with Dark Chocolate

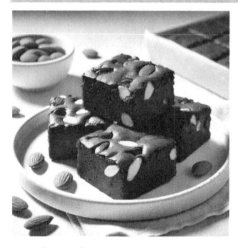

Number of servings: 9
Preparation time: 15 minutes
Cooking time: 25 minutes

Ingredients:

- 1 cup almond flour
- 1/2 cup unsweetened cocoa powder
- 1/2 cup dark chocolate chips
- 1/4 cup coconut oil, melted
- 1/4 cup maple syrup
- 2 large eggs
- 1 tsp vanilla extract
- 1/2 tsp baking powder
- Pinch of salt

Directions:

1. Preheat the oven to 350°F (175°C). Grease an 8x8-inch baking pan or line it with parchment paper.
2. In a large bowl, whisk together the almond flour, cocoa powder, baking powder, and salt.
3. Melt the coconut oil and thoroughly mix it with the maple syrup, eggs, and vanilla extract in a separate bowl.
4. After adding the wet components to the dry ingredients, mix just until incorporated.
5. Fold in the dark chocolate chips.
6. Pour the batter into the prepared baking pan and spread it evenly.
7. A toothpick inserted in the center should come out clean after baking for 20 to 25 minutes.
8. Let the brownies cool in the pan before cutting into 9 squares.

Nutritional value per serving:
Calories: 150, Carbs: 15g, Fiber: 3g, Sugars: 8g, Protein: 4g, Saturated fat: 6g, Unsaturated fat: 4g

Difficulty rating: ★★★☆☆

Tips for ingredient variations:
Add chopped nuts or a sprinkle of sea salt on top for extra crunch and flavor.

Lemon Sorbet with Mint

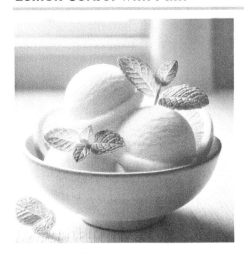

Number of servings: 4
Preparation time: 10 minutes
Freezing time: 4 hours

Ingredients:

- 1 cup squeezed lemon juice (4-6 lemons)
- 1 cup water
- 1/2 cup granulated sugar
- 1 tbsp fresh mint leaves, chopped

Directions:

1. Add the sugar and water to a small pot. Heat over medium heat, stirring occasionally, until the sugar is completely dissolved. Remove from heat and let cool.
2. Stir in the freshly squeezed lemon juice and chopped mint leaves.
3. Pour the mixture into a freezer-safe container and freeze for 4 hours, stirring every hour to break up any ice crystals.
4. Serve once the sorbet is fully frozen.

Nutritional value per serving: Calories: 110, Carbs: 28g, Fiber: 1g, Sugars: 25g, Protein: 0g, Saturated fat: 0g, Unsaturated fat: 0g

Difficulty rating: ★☆☆☆☆

Tips for ingredient variations: Add a teaspoon of lemon zest for an extra burst of flavor.

Pumpkin Protein Balls with Oats

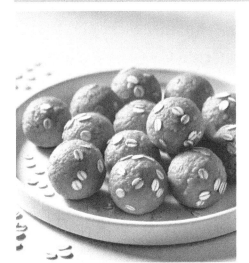

Number of servings: 10 (2 balls per serving)
Preparation time: 15 minutes

Ingredients:

- 1 cup rolled oats
- 1/2 cup pumpkin puree
- 1/4 cup almond butter
- 1/4 cup honey
- 1/4 cup vanilla protein powder
- 1 tsp pumpkin pie spice
- 1/2 tsp vanilla extract

Directions:

1. In a large bowl, combine the rolled oats, pumpkin puree, almond butter, honey, vanilla protein powder, pumpkin pie spice, and vanilla extract.
2. Mix until all ingredients are well combined.
3. Roll the mixture into small balls, about 1 inch in diameter.
4. Place the pumpkin protein balls on a baking sheet lined with parchment paper and refrigerate for at least 1 hour, or until firm.
5. For up to a week, keep in the refrigerator in an airtight container.

Nutritional value per serving: Calories: 120, Carbs: 18g, Fiber: 3g, Sugars: 10g, Protein: 5g, Saturated fat: 1g, Unsaturated fat: 5g

Difficulty rating: ★☆☆☆☆

Tips for ingredient variations: Add a handful of mini chocolate chips or chopped nuts for additional flavor and texture.

Coconut Macaroons with Dark Chocolate Drizzle

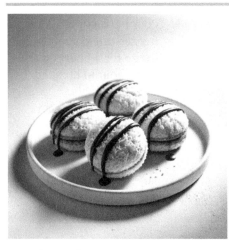

Number of servings: 12
Preparation time: 15 minutes
Cooking time: 25 minutes

Ingredients:

- 2 1/2 cups unsweetened shredded coconut
- 3 large egg whites
- 1/2 cup sugar
- 1 tsp vanilla extract
- 2 oz dark chocolate (70% cocoa or higher)

Directions:

1. Preheat the oven to 325°F (165°C). Line a baking sheet with parchment paper.
2. In a large bowl, mix together the shredded coconut, egg whites, sugar, and vanilla extract until well combined.
3. Using a tablespoon, scoop the mixture and form it into small mounds on the prepared baking sheet.
4. Bake for 20-25 minutes, or until the macaroons are golden brown.
5. Allow the macaroons to cool completely on the baking sheet.
6. Melt the dark chocolate in a microwave-safe bowl in 30-second intervals, stirring between each interval until smooth.
7. Drizzle the melted dark chocolate over the cooled macaroons.
8. Let the chocolate set before serving.

Nutritional value per serving: Calories: 140, Carbs: 12g, Fiber: 3g, Sugars: 9g, Protein: 2g, Saturated fat: 8g, Unsaturated fat: 2g

Difficulty rating: ★★☆☆☆

Tips for ingredient variations: Add a pinch of sea salt to the chocolate drizzle for a salted chocolate version.

Mixed Berry Parfait with Greek Yogurt and Granola

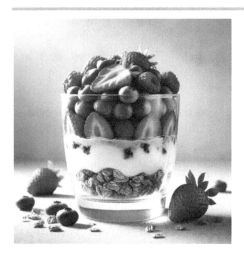

Number of servings: 1
Preparation time: 5 minutes

Ingredients:

- 1/2 cup Greek yogurt (low-fat)
- 1/2 cup of mixed berries (strawberries, raspberries, and blueberries)
- 2 tbsp granola
- 1 tsp honey (optional)

Directions:

1. Arrange half of the Greek yogurt in a bowl or serving glass.
2. Next, scatter half of the mixed berries over the yogurt.
3. Top the berries with 1 tablespoon of granola.
4. Repeat the layers with the remaining Greek yogurt, berries, and granola.
5. Drizzle with honey if desired.
6. Serve immediately.

Nutritional value per serving: Calories: 130, Carbs: 20g, Fiber: 3g, Sugars: 12g, Protein: 8g, Saturated fat: 1g, Unsaturated fat: 1g

Difficulty rating: ★☆☆☆☆

Tips for ingredient variations: Substitute the mixed berries with any seasonal fruit or a combination of your favorites.

Low-Calorie Cheesecake Bites with Berry Sauce

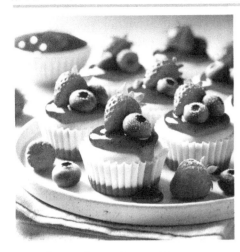

Number of servings: 12
Preparation time: 20 minutes
Cooking time: 20 minutes (plus chilling time)

Ingredients:

- 8 oz low-fat cream cheese
- 1/4 cup Greek yogurt (low-fat)
- 1/4 cup sugar
- 1 tsp vanilla extract
- 1 large egg
- 1 cup of mixed berries (strawberries, raspberries, and blueberries)
- 1 tbsp honey

Directions:

1. Preheat the oven to 350°F (175°C). Line a mini muffin tin with paper liners.
2. In a medium bowl, beat the cream cheese, Greek yogurt, sugar, and vanilla extract until smooth.
3. Add the egg and mix until well combined.
4. Divide the mixture evenly among the prepared muffin cups.
5. Bake for 15-20 minutes, or until the centers are set.
6. Let the cheesecake bites cool completely, then refrigerate for at least 2 hours.
7. In a small saucepan, combine the mixed berries and honey. Simmer for 5 to 7 minutes over medium heat, or until the berries soften and the sauce thickens.
8. Spoon the berry sauce over the chilled cheesecake bites before serving.

Nutritional value per serving: Calories: 150, Carbs: 18g, Fiber: 2g, Sugars: 14g, Protein: 4g, Saturated fat: 3g, Unsaturated fat: 2g

Difficulty rating: ★★☆☆☆

Tips for ingredient variations: Use a variety of berries for the sauce to add different flavors and colors.

Peach Yogurt Popsicles with Honey

Number of servings: 6
Preparation time: 10 minutes

Freezing time: 4 hours

Ingredients:

- 2 cups Greek yogurt (low-fat)
- 2 ripe peaches, peeled and diced
- 2 tbsp honey
- 1 tsp vanilla extract

Directions:

1. In a blender, combine the Greek yogurt, diced peaches, honey, and vanilla extract. Blend until smooth.
2. Pour the mixture into popsicle molds.
3. Put the popsicle sticks in and freeze for four hours or until the popsicles are hardened.
4. Put the molds under warm water for a brief period of time to release the popsicles.
5. Serve immediately.

Nutritional value per serving: Calories: 110, Carbs: 18g, Fiber: 1g, Sugars: 16g, Protein: 5g, Saturated fat: 0g, Unsaturated fat: 0g

Difficulty rating: ★☆☆☆☆

Tips for ingredient variations: Substitute peaches with other fruits such as mangoes or strawberries for different flavor popsicles.

Strawberry Banana Smoothie with Almond Milk

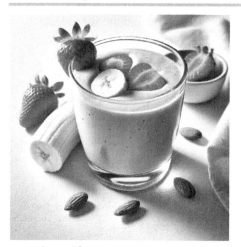

Number of servings: 1

Preparation time: 5 minutes

Ingredients:

- 1 cup almond milk (unsweetened)
- 1/2 cup strawberries, hulled
- 1 small banana
- 1 tbsp chia seeds
- 1 tsp honey (optional)

Directions:

1. In a blender, combine the almond milk, strawberries, banana, chia seeds, and honey if using.
2. Blend until smooth and creamy.
3. Pour into a glass and serve immediately.

Nutritional value per serving: Calories: 140, Carbs: 29g, Fiber: 7g, Sugars: 18g, Protein: 3g, Saturated fat: 0g, Unsaturated fat: 2g

Difficulty rating: ★☆☆☆

Tips for ingredient variations: Add a handful of spinach for an extra nutrient boost without altering the flavor significantly.

60-DAY MEAL PLAN

This meal plan is designed to help you embrace a nutritious and balanced diet, inspired by the effective principles of Dr. Nowzaradan. Each day, you will enjoy delicious, satisfying meals that support your weight loss goals and overall wellness. Remember that progress, not perfection, is the goal of this trip. Every healthy choice you make brings you one step closer to the vibrant, energetic life you deserve. Stay committed, stay positive, and let this meal plan guide you towards a healthier, happier you. You've got this!

Day 1

- **Breakfast**: Greek Yogurt with Berries and Honey - 200 calories
- **Lunch**: Grilled Chicken Breast with Steamed Broccoli and Quinoa - 350 calories
- **Side**: Garlic Green Beans with Almonds - 60 calories
- **Dinner**: Baked Salmon with Asparagus and Brown Rice - 380 calories
- **Side**: Cucumber and Tomato Salad with Feta - 60 calories
- **Dessert**: Frozen Yogurt Bark with Berries and Nuts - 120 calories
- **Total**: 1170 calories

Day 2

- **Breakfast**: Scrambled Egg Whites with Spinach and Feta - 150 calories
- **Lunch**: Turkey Meatballs with Zucchini Noodles and Marinara Sauce - 320 calories
- **Side**: Roasted Brussels Sprouts with Balsamic Glaze - 70 calories
- **Dinner**: Chicken and Vegetable Soup with Barley - 300 calories
- **Side**: Mashed Cauliflower with Garlic - 70 calories

- **Dessert**: Chocolate Avocado Pudding with Berries - 150 calories
- **Total**: 1060 calories

Day 3

- **Breakfast**: Oatmeal with Almond Milk, Blueberries, and Chia Seeds - 220 calories
- **Lunch**: Quinoa Salad with Chickpeas, Veggies, and Feta - 380 calories
- **Side**: Steamed Snap Peas with Sesame Seeds - 50 calories
- **Dinner**: Baked Cod with Lemon, Dill, and Wild Rice - 320 calories
- **Side**: Tomato Basil Salad with Mozzarella - 50 calories
- **Dessert**: Baked Apples with Cinnamon and Walnuts - 120 calories
- **Total**: 1140 calories

Day 4

- **Breakfast**: Protein Smoothie (Spinach, Banana, Almond Milk, Protein Powder) - 250 calories
- **Lunch**: Stir-Fried Vegetables with Brown Rice and Tofu - 350 calories
- **Side**: Roasted Butternut Squash with Cinnamon - 100 calories

- **Dinner**: Chicken Fajitas with Bell Peppers, Onions, and Whole Wheat Tortilla - 350 calories
- **Side**: Mixed Greens with Balsamic Vinaigrette and Walnuts - 70 calories
- **Dessert**: Chia Seed Pudding with Mango and Coconut Milk - 140 calories
- **Total**: 1260 calories

Day 5

- **Breakfast**: Whole Wheat Toast with Avocado and Tomato - 200 calories
- **Lunch**: Grilled Shrimp Skewers with Bell Peppers and Couscous - 330 calories
- **Side**: Garlic Green Beans with Almonds - 60 calories
- **Dinner**: Stir-fried Broccoli and Beef with Brown Rice - 380 calories
- **Side**: Sauteed Spinach with Garlic and Olive Oil - 60 calories
- **Dessert**: Greek Yogurt with Honey, Walnuts, and Blueberries - 150 calories
- **Total**: 1180 calories

Day 6

- **Breakfast**: Cottage Cheese with Pineapple and Almonds - 180 calories

- **Lunch**: Black Bean and Corn Salad with Avocado - 300 calories
- **Side**: Baked Sweet Potato Fries with Paprika - 100 calories
- **Dinner**: Zucchini Lasagna with Ground Turkey - 380 calories
- **Side**: Sauteed Mushrooms with Thyme - 60 calories
- **Dessert**: Fruit Salad with Mint and Lime - 90 calories
- **Total**: 1110 calories

Day 7

- **Breakfast**: Boiled Eggs and Sliced Avocado - 200 calories
- **Lunch**: Turkey and Avocado Lettuce Wraps with Salsa - 280 calories
- **Side**: Cucumber and Tomato Salad with Feta - 60 calories
- **Dinner**: Grilled Chicken with Cauliflower Mash and Green Beans - 320 calories
- **Side**: Roasted Carrots with Thyme and Honey - 80 calories
- **Dessert**: Banana Ice Cream with Dark Chocolate - 130 calories
- **Total**: 1070 calories

Day 8

- **Breakfast**: Apple Slices with Almond Butter and Cinnamon - 220 calories
- **Lunch**: Vegetarian Chili with Quinoa - 330 calories
- **Side**: Garlic Green Beans with Almonds - 60 calories
- **Dinner**: Grilled Tuna with Mixed Greens and Quinoa - 320 calories

- **Side**: Sauteed Spinach with Garlic and Olive Oil - 60 calories
- **Dessert**: Almond Flour Brownies with Dark Chocolate - 150 calories
- **Total**: 1140 calories

Day 9

- **Breakfast**: Vegetable Omelette (Egg Whites, Bell Peppers, Onions, Mushrooms) - 200 calories
- **Lunch**: Stuffed Bell Peppers with Ground Turkey and Brown Rice - 340 calories
- **Side**: Steamed Snap Peas with Sesame Seeds - 50 calories
- **Dinner**: Baked Eggplant Parmesan with Marinara Sauce - 340 calories
- **Side**: Mixed Greens with Balsamic Vinaigrette and Walnuts - 70 calories
- **Dessert**: Lemon Sorbet with Mint - 110 calories
- **Total**: 1110 calories

Day 10

- **Breakfast**: Low-Fat Cheese and Turkey Bacon - 200 calories
- **Lunch**: Chicken and Black Bean Burrito Bowl with Brown Rice - 380 calories
- **Side**: Tomato Basil Salad with Mozzarella - 50 calories
- **Dinner**: Beef and Vegetable Kebabs with Quinoa - 350 calories
- **Side**: Sauteed Mushrooms with Thyme - 60 calories
- **Dessert**: Pumpkin Protein Balls with Oats - 120 calories
- **Total**: 1160 calories

Day 11

- **Breakfast**: Chia Seed Pudding with Almond Milk, Strawberries, and Nuts - 230 calories
- **Lunch**: Quinoa Salad with Chickpeas, Veggies, and Feta - 380 calories
- **Side**: Roasted Brussels Sprouts with Balsamic Glaze - 70 calories
- **Dinner**: Chicken Stir-Fry with Brown Rice and Veggies - 380 calories
- **Side**: Garlic Green Beans with Almonds - 60 calories
- **Dessert**: Coconut Macaroons with Dark Chocolate Drizzle - 140 calories
- **Total**: 1260 calories

Day 12

- **Breakfast**: Quinoa Porridge with Almonds and Honey - 250 calories
- **Lunch**: Grilled Shrimp Skewers with Bell Peppers and Couscous - 330 calories
- **Side**: Steamed Snap Peas with Sesame Seeds - 50 calories
- **Dinner**: Cabbage Rolls with Ground Turkey and Brown Rice - 340 calories
- **Side**: Sauteed Spinach with Garlic and Olive Oil - 60 calories
- **Dessert**: Mixed Berry Parfait with Greek Yogurt and Granola - 130 calories
- **Total**: 1160 calories

Day 13

- **Breakfast**: Smoothie Bowl (Berries, Spinach, Almond Milk, Protein Powder, Granola) - 280 calories

- **Lunch**: Black Bean and Corn Salad with Avocado - 300 calories
- **Side**: Baked Sweet Potato Fries with Paprika - 100 calories
- **Dinner**: Turkey and Spinach Stuffed Mushrooms with Cheese - 300 calories
- **Side**: Sauteed Mushrooms with Thyme - 60 calories
- **Dessert**: Low-Calorie Cheesecake Bites with Berry Sauce - 150 calories
- **Total**: 1190 calories

Day 14

- **Breakfast**: Low-Fat Greek Yogurt with Granola and Berries - 220 calories
- **Lunch**: Chicken and Vegetable Soup with Barley - 300 calories
- **Side**: Roasted Butternut Squash with Cinnamon - 100 calories
- **Dinner**: Spaghetti Squash with Turkey Bolognese and Parmesan - 330 calories
- **Side**: Garlic Green Beans with Almonds - 60 calories
- **Dessert**: Peach Yogurt Popsicles with Honey - 110 calories
- **Total**: 1120 calories

Day 15

- **Breakfast**: Breakfast Burrito (Egg Whites, Spinach, Whole Wheat Tortilla, Salsa) - 250 calories
- **Lunch**: Grilled Chicken Breast with Steamed Broccoli and Quinoa - 350 calories

- **Side**: Steamed Snap Peas with Sesame Seeds - 50 calories
- **Dinner**: Chicken Caesar Salad (Light Dressing, Whole Wheat Croutons) - 300 calories
- **Side**: Sauteed Spinach with Garlic and Olive Oil - 60 calories
- **Dessert**: Strawberry Banana Smoothie with Almond Milk - 140 calories
- **Total**: 1150 calories

Day 16

- **Breakfast**: Pumpkin Spice Oatmeal with Walnuts - 220 calories
- **Lunch**: Stir-fried Broccoli and Beef with Brown Rice - 380 calories
- **Side**: Roasted Brussels Sprouts with Balsamic Glaze - 70 calories
- **Dinner**: Grilled Tuna with Mixed Greens and Quinoa - 320 calories
- **Side**: Garlic Green Beans with Almonds - 60 calories
- **Dessert**: Frozen Yogurt Bark with Berries and Nuts - 120 calories
- **Total**: 1170 calories

Day 17

- **Breakfast**: Banana Protein Pancakes with Maple Syrup - 250 calories
- **Lunch**: Stir-Fried Vegetables with Brown Rice and Tofu - 350 calories
- **Side**: Mixed Greens with Balsamic Vinaigrette and Walnuts - 70 calories
- **Dinner**: Zucchini Lasagna with Ground Turkey - 380 calories

- **Side**: Roasted Carrots with Thyme and Honey - 80 calories
- **Dessert**: Chocolate Avocado Pudding with Berries - 150 calories
- **Total**: 1200 calories

Day 18

- **Breakfast**: Tomato and Avocado Salad with Olive Oil - 200 calories
- **Lunch**: Grilled Shrimp Skewers with Bell Peppers and Couscous - 330 calories
- **Side**: Steamed Snap Peas with Sesame Seeds - 50 calories
- **Dinner**: Chicken Fajitas with Bell Peppers, Onions, and Whole Wheat Tortilla - 350 calories
- **Side**: Garlic Green Beans with Almonds - 60 calories
- **Dessert**: Greek Yogurt with Honey, Walnuts, and Blueberries - 150 calories
- **Total**: 1140 calories

Day 19

- **Breakfast**: Spinach and Mushroom Frittata with Cheese - 220 calories
- **Lunch**: Turkey Meatballs with Zucchini Noodles and Marinara Sauce - 320 calories
- **Side**: Roasted Brussels Sprouts with Balsamic Glaze - 70 calories
- **Dinner**: Beef and Vegetable Kebabs with Quinoa - 350 calories
- **Side**: Sauteed Mushrooms with Thyme - 60 calories
- **Dessert**: Baked Apples with Cinnamon and Walnuts - 120 calories
- **Total**: 1140 calories

Day 20

- **Breakfast**: Berry and Almond Smoothie - 230 calories
- **Lunch**: Black Bean and Corn Salad with Avocado - 300 calories
- **Side**: Baked Sweet Potato Fries with Paprika - 100 calories
- **Dinner**: Cabbage Rolls with Ground Turkey and Brown Rice - 340 calories
- **Side**: Sauteed Spinach with Garlic and Olive Oil - 60 calories
- **Dessert**: Chia Seed Pudding with Mango and Coconut Milk - 140 calories
- **Total**: 1170 calories

Day 21

- **Breakfast**: Peanut Butter Banana Toast with Chia Seeds - 220 calories
- **Lunch**: Chicken and Vegetable Soup with Barley - 300 calories
- **Side**: Steamed Snap Peas with Sesame Seeds - 50 calories
- **Dinner**: Grilled Chicken with Cauliflower Mash and Green Beans - 320 calories
- **Side**: Tomato Basil Salad with Mozzarella - 50 calories
- **Dessert**: Greek Yogurt with Honey, Walnuts, and Blueberries - 150 calories
- **Total**: 1090 calories

Day 22

- **Breakfast**: Mixed Fruit Salad with Greek Yogurt - 200 calories
- **Lunch**: Stir-Fried Vegetables with Brown Rice and Tofu - 350 calories

- **Side**: Garlic Green Beans with Almonds - 60 calories
- **Dinner**: Baked Eggplant Parmesan with Marinara Sauce - 340 calories
- **Side**: Sauteed Mushrooms with Thyme - 60 calories
- **Dessert**: Lemon Sorbet with Mint - 110 calories
- **Total**: 1120 calories

Day 23

- **Breakfast**: Zucchini Bread with Cream Cheese - 220 calories
- **Lunch**: Quinoa Salad with Chickpeas, Veggies, and Feta - 380 calories
- **Side**: Roasted Brussels Sprouts with Balsamic Glaze - 70 calories
- **Dinner**: Grilled Tuna with Mixed Greens and Quinoa - 320 calories
- **Side**: Sauteed Spinach with Garlic and Olive Oil - 60 calories
- **Dessert**: Frozen Yogurt Bark with Berries and Nuts - 120 calories
- **Total**: 1170 calories

Day 24

- **Breakfast**: Almond Butter and Banana Smoothie with Protein Powder - 250 calories
- **Lunch**: Black Bean and Corn Salad with Avocado - 300 calories
- **Side**: Baked Sweet Potato Fries with Paprika - 100 calories
- **Dinner**: Zucchini Lasagna with Ground Turkey - 380 calories
- **Side**: Sauteed Mushrooms with Thyme - 60 calories
- **Dessert**: Mixed Berry Parfait with Greek Yogurt and Granola - 130 calories

- **Total**: 1220 calories

Day 25

- **Breakfast**: Egg Muffins with Veggies and Cheese - 200 calories
- **Lunch**: Grilled Chicken Breast with Steamed Broccoli and Quinoa - 350 calories
- **Side**: Steamed Snap Peas with Sesame Seeds - 50 calories
- **Dinner**: Stir-fried Broccoli and Beef with Brown Rice - 380 calories
- **Side**: Garlic Green Beans with Almonds - 60 calories
- **Dessert**: Chocolate Avocado Pudding with Berries - 150 calories
- **Total**: 1190 calories

Day 26

- **Breakfast**: Tropical Smoothie (Mango, Pineapple, Coconut Milk, Chia Seeds) - 230 calories
- **Lunch**: Chicken Caesar Salad (Light Dressing, Whole Wheat Croutons) - 300 calories
- **Side**: Garlic Green Beans with Almonds - 60 calories
- **Dinner**: Cabbage Rolls with Ground Turkey and Brown Rice - 340 calories
- **Side**: Roasted Brussels Sprouts with Balsamic Glaze - 70 calories
- **Dessert**: Greek Yogurt with Honey, Walnuts, and Blueberries - 150 calories
- **Total**: 1150 calories

Day 27

- **Breakfast**: Oatmeal with Chia Seeds, Fresh Berries, and Almonds - 230 calories

- **Lunch**: Turkey Meatballs with Zucchini Noodles and Marinara Sauce - 320 calories
- **Side**: Steamed Snap Peas with Sesame Seeds - 50 calories
- **Dinner**: Chicken Fajitas with Bell Peppers, Onions, and Whole Wheat Tortilla - 350 calories
- **Side**: Sauteed Mushrooms with Thyme - 60 calories
- **Dessert**: Coconut Macaroons with Dark Chocolate Drizzle - 140 calories
- **Total**: 1150 calories

Day 28

- **Breakfast**: Turkey Sausage and Veggie Scramble - 250 calories
- **Lunch**: Quinoa Salad with Chickpeas, Veggies, and Feta - 380 calories
- **Side**: Roasted Brussels Sprouts with Balsamic Glaze - 70 calories
- **Dinner**: Beef and Vegetable Kebabs with Quinoa - 350 calories
- **Side**: Garlic Green Beans with Almonds - 60 calories
- **Dessert**: Pumpkin Protein Balls with Oats - 120 calories
- **Total**: 1230 calories

Day 29

- **Breakfast**: Ricotta Cheese with Fresh Berries and Honey - 200 calories
- **Lunch**: Black Bean and Corn Salad with Avocado - 300 calories
- **Side**: Baked Sweet Potato Fries with Paprika - 100 calories

- **Dinner**: Zucchini Lasagna with Ground Turkey - 380 calories
- **Side**: Sauteed Spinach with Garlic and Olive Oil - 60 calories
- **Dessert**: Mixed Berry Parfait with Greek Yogurt and Granola - 130 calories
- **Total**: 1170 calories

Day 30

- **Breakfast**: Low-Carb Breakfast Wrap (Lettuce, Turkey, Cheese, Avocado) - 220 calories
- **Lunch**: Chicken and Black Bean Burrito Bowl with Brown Rice - 380 calories
- **Side**: Tomato Basil Salad with Mozzarella - 50 calories
- **Dinner**: Grilled Tuna with Mixed Greens and Quinoa - 320 calories
- **Side**: Garlic Green Beans with Almonds - 60 calories
- **Dessert**: Frozen Yogurt Bark with Berries and Nuts - 120 calories
- **Total**: 1150 calories

Day 31

- **Breakfast**: Greek Yogurt with Berries and Honey - 200 calories
- **Lunch**: Grilled Chicken Breast with Steamed Broccoli and Quinoa - 350 calories
- **Side**: Garlic Green Beans with Almonds - 60 calories
- **Dinner**: Baked Salmon with Asparagus and Brown Rice - 380 calories
- **Side**: Cucumber and Tomato Salad with Feta - 60 calories

- **Dessert**: Frozen Yogurt Bark with Berries and Nuts - 120 calories
- **Total**: 1170 calories

Day 32

- **Breakfast**: Scrambled Egg Whites with Spinach and Feta - 150 calories
- **Lunch**: Turkey Meatballs with Zucchini Noodles and Marinara Sauce - 320 calories
- **Side**: Roasted Brussels Sprouts with Balsamic Glaze - 70 calories
- **Dinner**: Chicken and Vegetable Soup with Barley - 300 calories
- **Side**: Mashed Cauliflower with Garlic - 70 calories
- **Dessert**: Chocolate Avocado Pudding with Berries - 150 calories
- **Total**: 1060 calories

Day 33

- **Breakfast**: Oatmeal with Almond Milk, Blueberries, and Chia Seeds - 220 calories
- **Lunch**: Quinoa Salad with Chickpeas, Veggies, and Feta - 380 calories
- **Side**: Steamed Snap Peas with Sesame Seeds - 50 calories
- **Dinner**: Baked Cod with Lemon, Dill, and Wild Rice - 320 calories
- **Side**: Tomato Basil Salad with Mozzarella - 50 calories
- **Dessert**: Baked Apples with Cinnamon and Walnuts - 120 calories
- **Total**: 1140 calories

Day 34

- **Breakfast**: Protein Smoothie (Spinach, Banana, Almond Milk,

Protein Powder) - 250 calories
- **Lunch**: Stir-Fried Vegetables with Brown Rice and Tofu - 350 calories
- **Side**: Roasted Butternut Squash with Cinnamon - 100 calories
- **Dinner**: Chicken Fajitas with Bell Peppers, Onions, and Whole Wheat Tortilla - 350 calories
- **Side**: Mixed Greens with Balsamic Vinaigrette and Walnuts - 70 calories
- **Dessert**: Chia Seed Pudding with Mango and Coconut Milk - 140 calories
- **Total**: 1260 calories

Day 35

- **Breakfast**: Whole Wheat Toast with Avocado and Tomato - 200 calories
- **Lunch**: Grilled Shrimp Skewers with Bell Peppers and Couscous - 330 calories
- **Side**: Garlic Green Beans with Almonds - 60 calories
- **Dinner**: Stir-fried Broccoli and Beef with Brown Rice - 380 calories
- **Side**: Sauteed Spinach with Garlic and Olive Oil - 60 calories
- **Dessert**: Greek Yogurt with Honey, Walnuts, and Blueberries - 150 calories
- **Total**: 1180 calories

Day 36

- **Breakfast**: Cottage Cheese with Pineapple and Almonds - 180 calories
- **Lunch**: Black Bean and Corn Salad with Avocado - 300 calories

- **Side**: Baked Sweet Potato Fries with Paprika - 100 calories
- **Dinner**: Zucchini Lasagna with Ground Turkey - 380 calories
- **Side**: Sauteed Mushrooms with Thyme - 60 calories
- **Dessert**: Fruit Salad with Mint and Lime - 90 calories
- **Total**: 1110 calories

Day 37

- **Breakfast**: Boiled Eggs and Sliced Avocado - 200 calories
- **Lunch**: Turkey and Avocado Lettuce Wraps with Salsa - 280 calories
- **Side**: Cucumber and Tomato Salad with Feta - 60 calories
- **Dinner**: Grilled Chicken with Cauliflower Mash and Green Beans - 320 calories
- **Side**: Roasted Carrots with Thyme and Honey - 80 calories
- **Dessert**: Banana Ice Cream with Dark Chocolate - 130 calories
- **Total**: 1070 calories

Day 38

- **Breakfast**: Apple Slices with Almond Butter and Cinnamon - 220 calories
- **Lunch**: Vegetarian Chili with Quinoa - 330 calories
- **Side**: Garlic Green Beans with Almonds - 60 calories
- **Dinner**: Grilled Tuna with Mixed Greens and Quinoa - 320 calories
- **Side**: Sauteed Spinach with Garlic and Olive Oil - 60 calories

- **Dessert**: Almond Flour Brownies with Dark Chocolate - 150 calories
- **Total**: 1140 calories

Day 39

- **Breakfast**: Vegetable Omelette (Egg Whites, Bell Peppers, Onions, Mushrooms) - 200 calories
- **Lunch**: Stuffed Bell Peppers with Ground Turkey and Brown Rice - 340 calories
- **Side**: Steamed Snap Peas with Sesame Seeds - 50 calories
- **Dinner**: Baked Eggplant Parmesan with Marinara Sauce - 340 calories
- **Side**: Mixed Greens with Balsamic Vinaigrette and Walnuts - 70 calories
- **Dessert**: Lemon Sorbet with Mint - 110 calories
- **Total**: 1110 calories

Day 40

- **Breakfast**: Low-Fat Cheese and Turkey Bacon - 200 calories
- **Lunch**: Chicken and Black Bean Burrito Bowl with Brown Rice - 380 calories
- **Side**: Tomato Basil Salad with Mozzarella - 50 calories
- **Dinner**: Beef and Vegetable Kebabs with Quinoa - 350 calories
- **Side**: Sauteed Mushrooms with Thyme - 60 calories
- **Dessert**: Pumpkin Protein Balls with Oats - 120 calories
- **Total**: 1160 calories

Day 41

- **Breakfast**: Chia Seed Pudding with Almond

80 The Dr. Now 1200-Calorie Diet Plan

Milk, Strawberries, and Nuts - 230 calories
- **Lunch**: Quinoa Salad with Chickpeas, Veggies, and Feta - 380 calories
- **Side**: Roasted Brussels Sprouts with Balsamic Glaze - 70 calories
- **Dinner**: Chicken Stir-Fry with Brown Rice and Veggies - 380 calories
- **Side**: Garlic Green Beans with Almonds - 60 calories
- **Dessert**: Coconut Macaroons with Dark Chocolate Drizzle - 140 calories
- **Total**: 1260 calories

Day 42

- **Breakfast**: Quinoa Porridge with Almonds and Honey - 250 calories
- **Lunch**: Grilled Shrimp Skewers with Bell Peppers and Couscous - 330 calories
- **Side**: Steamed Snap Peas with Sesame Seeds - 50 calories
- **Dinner**: Cabbage Rolls with Ground Turkey and Brown Rice - 340 calories
- **Side**: Sauteed Spinach with Garlic and Olive Oil - 60 calories
- **Dessert**: Mixed Berry Parfait with Greek Yogurt and Granola - 130 calories
- **Total**: 1160 calories

Day 43

- **Breakfast**: Smoothie Bowl (Berries, Spinach, Almond Milk, Protein Powder, Granola) - 280 calories
- **Lunch**: Black Bean and Corn Salad with Avocado - 300 calories

- **Side**: Baked Sweet Potato Fries with Paprika - 100 calories
- **Dinner**: Turkey and Spinach Stuffed Mushrooms with Cheese - 300 calories
- **Side**: Sauteed Mushrooms with Thyme - 60 calories
- **Dessert**: Low-Calorie Cheesecake Bites with Berry Sauce - 150 calories
- **Total**: 1190 calories

Day 44

- **Breakfast**: Low-Fat Greek Yogurt with Granola and Berries - 220 calories
- **Lunch**: Chicken and Vegetable Soup with Barley - 300 calories
- **Side**: Roasted Butternut Squash with Cinnamon - 100 calories
- **Dinner**: Spaghetti Squash with Turkey Bolognese and Parmesan - 330 calories
- **Side**: Garlic Green Beans with Almonds - 60 calories
- **Dessert**: Peach Yogurt Popsicles with Honey - 110 calories
- **Total**: 1120 calories

Day 45

- **Breakfast**: Breakfast Burrito (Egg Whites, Spinach, Whole Wheat Tortilla, Salsa) - 250 calories
- **Lunch**: Grilled Chicken Breast with Steamed Broccoli and Quinoa - 350 calories
- **Side**: Steamed Snap Peas with Sesame Seeds - 50 calories
- **Dinner**: Chicken Caesar Salad (Light Dressing,

Whole Wheat Croutons) - 300 calories
- **Side**: Sauteed Spinach with Garlic and Olive Oil - 60 calories
- **Dessert**: Strawberry Banana Smoothie with Almond Milk - 140 calories
- **Total**: 1150 calories

Day 46

- **Breakfast**: Pumpkin Spice Oatmeal with Walnuts - 220 calories
- **Lunch**: Stir-fried Broccoli and Beef with Brown Rice - 380 calories
- **Side**: Roasted Brussels Sprouts with Balsamic Glaze - 70 calories
- **Dinner**: Grilled Tuna with Mixed Greens and Quinoa - 320 calories
- **Side**: Garlic Green Beans with Almonds - 60 calories
- **Dessert**: Frozen Yogurt Bark with Berries and Nuts - 120 calories
- **Total**: 1170 calories

Day 47

- **Breakfast**: Banana Protein Pancakes with Maple Syrup - 250 calories
- **Lunch**: Stir-Fried Vegetables with Brown Rice and Tofu - 350 calories
- **Side**: Mixed Greens with Balsamic Vinaigrette and Walnuts - 70 calories
- **Dinner**: Zucchini Lasagna with Ground Turkey - 380 calories
- **Side**: Roasted Carrots with Thyme and Honey - 80 calories
- **Dessert**: Chocolate Avocado Pudding with Berries - 150 calories

- **Total**: 1200 calories

Day 48

- **Breakfast**: Tomato and Avocado Salad with Olive Oil - 200 calories
- **Lunch**: Grilled Shrimp Skewers with Bell Peppers and Couscous - 330 calories
- **Side**: Steamed Snap Peas with Sesame Seeds - 50 calories
- **Dinner**: Chicken Fajitas with Bell Peppers, Onions, and Whole Wheat Tortilla - 350 calories
- **Side**: Garlic Green Beans with Almonds - 60 calories
- **Dessert**: Greek Yogurt with Honey, Walnuts, and Blueberries - 150 calories
- **Total**: 1140 calories

Day 49

- **Breakfast**: Spinach and Mushroom Frittata with Cheese - 220 calories
- **Lunch**: Turkey Meatballs with Zucchini Noodles and Marinara Sauce - 320 calories
- **Side**: Roasted Brussels Sprouts with Balsamic Glaze - 70 calories
- **Dinner**: Beef and Vegetable Kebabs with Quinoa - 350 calories
- **Side**: Sauteed Mushrooms with Thyme - 60 calories
- **Dessert**: Baked Apples with Cinnamon and Walnuts - 120 calories
- **Total**: 1140 calories

Day 50

- **Breakfast**: Berry and Almond Smoothie - 230 calories

- **Lunch**: Black Bean and Corn Salad with Avocado - 300 calories
- **Side**: Baked Sweet Potato Fries with Paprika - 100 calories
- **Dinner**: Cabbage Rolls with Ground Turkey and Brown Rice - 340 calories
- **Side**: Sauteed Spinach with Garlic and Olive Oil - 60 calories
- **Dessert**: Chia Seed Pudding with Mango and Coconut Milk - 140 calories
- **Total**: 1170 calories

Day 51

- **Breakfast**: Peanut Butter Banana Toast with Chia Seeds - 220 calories
- **Lunch**: Chicken and Vegetable Soup with Barley - 300 calories
- **Side**: Steamed Snap Peas with Sesame Seeds - 50 calories
- **Dinner**: Grilled Chicken with Cauliflower Mash and Green Beans - 320 calories
- **Side**: Tomato Basil Salad with Mozzarella - 50 calories
- **Dessert**: Greek Yogurt with Honey, Walnuts, and Blueberries - 150 calories
- **Total**: 1090 calories

Day 52

- **Breakfast**: Mixed Fruit Salad with Greek Yogurt - 200 calories
- **Lunch**: Stir-Fried Vegetables with Brown Rice and Tofu - 350 calories
- **Side**: Garlic Green Beans with Almonds - 60 calories

- **Dinner**: Baked Eggplant Parmesan with Marinara Sauce - 340 calories
- **Side**: Sauteed Mushrooms with Thyme - 60 calories
- **Dessert**: Lemon Sorbet with Mint - 110 calories
- **Total**: 1120 calories

Day 53

- **Breakfast**: Zucchini Bread with Cream Cheese - 220 calories
- **Lunch**: Quinoa Salad with Chickpeas, Veggies, and Feta - 380 calories
- **Side**: Roasted Brussels Sprouts with Balsamic Glaze - 70 calories
- **Dinner**: Grilled Tuna with Mixed Greens and Quinoa - 320 calories
- **Side**: Sauteed Spinach with Garlic and Olive Oil - 60 calories
- **Dessert**: Frozen Yogurt Bark with Berries and Nuts - 120 calories
- **Total**: 1170 calories

Day 54

- **Breakfast**: Almond Butter and Banana Smoothie with Protein Powder - 250 calories
- **Lunch**: Black Bean and Corn Salad with Avocado - 300 calories
- **Side**: Baked Sweet Potato Fries with Paprika - 100 calories
- **Dinner**: Zucchini Lasagna with Ground Turkey - 380 calories
- **Side**: Sauteed Mushrooms with Thyme - 60 calories
- **Dessert**: Mixed Berry Parfait with Greek Yogurt and Granola - 130 calories
- **Total**: 1220 calories

Day 55

- **Breakfast**: Egg Muffins with Veggies and Cheese - 200 calories
- **Lunch**: Grilled Chicken Breast with Steamed Broccoli and Quinoa - 350 calories
- **Side**: Steamed Snap Peas with Sesame Seeds - 50 calories
- **Dinner**: Stir-fried Broccoli and Beef with Brown Rice - 380 calories
- **Side**: Garlic Green Beans with Almonds - 60 calories
- **Dessert**: Chocolate Avocado Pudding with Berries - 150 calories
- **Total**: 1190 calories

Day 56

- **Breakfast**: Tropical Smoothie (Mango, Pineapple, Coconut Milk, Chia Seeds) - 230 calories
- **Lunch**: Chicken Caesar Salad (Light Dressing, Whole Wheat Croutons) - 300 calories
- **Side**: Garlic Green Beans with Almonds - 60 calories
- **Dinner**: Cabbage Rolls with Ground Turkey and Brown Rice - 340 calories
- **Side**: Roasted Brussels Sprouts with Balsamic Glaze - 70 calories
- **Dessert**: Greek Yogurt with Honey, Walnuts, and Blueberries - 150 calories
- **Total**: 1150 calories

Day 57

- **Breakfast**: Oatmeal with Chia Seeds, Fresh Berries, and Almonds - 230 calories
- **Lunch**: Turkey Meatballs with Zucchini Noodles and Marinara Sauce - 320 calories
- **Side**: Steamed Snap Peas with Sesame Seeds - 50 calories
- **Dinner**: Chicken Fajitas with Bell Peppers, Onions, and Whole Wheat Tortilla - 350 calories
- **Side**: Sauteed Mushrooms with Thyme - 60 calories
- **Dessert**: Coconut Macaroons with Dark Chocolate Drizzle - 140 calories
- **Total**: 1150 calories

Day 58

- **Breakfast**: Turkey Sausage and Veggie Scramble - 250 calories
- **Lunch**: Quinoa Salad with Chickpeas, Veggies, and Feta - 380 calories
- **Side**: Roasted Brussels Sprouts with Balsamic Glaze - 70 calories
- **Dinner**: Beef and Vegetable Kebabs with Quinoa - 350 calories
- **Side**: Garlic Green Beans with Almonds - 60 calories
- **Dessert**: Pumpkin Protein Balls with Oats - 120 calories
- **Total**: 1230 calories

Day 59

- **Breakfast**: Ricotta Cheese with Fresh Berries and Honey - 200 calories
- **Lunch**: Black Bean and Corn Salad with Avocado - 300 calories
- **Side**: Baked Sweet Potato Fries with Paprika - 100 calories
- **Dinner**: Zucchini Lasagna with Ground Turkey - 380 calories
- **Side**: Sauteed Spinach with Garlic and Olive Oil - 60 calories
- **Dessert**: Mixed Berry Parfait with Greek Yogurt and Granola - 130 calories
- **Total**: 1170 calories

Day 60

- **Breakfast**: Low-Carb Breakfast Wrap (Lettuce, Turkey, Cheese, Avocado) - 220 calories
- **Lunch**: Chicken and Black Bean Burrito Bowl with Brown Rice - 380 calories
- **Side**: Tomato Basil Salad with Mozzarella - 50 calories
- **Dinner**: Grilled Tuna with Mixed Greens and Quinoa - 320 calories
- **Side**: Garlic Green Beans with Almonds - 60 calories
- **Dessert**: Frozen Yogurt Bark with Berries and Nuts - 120 calories
- **Total**: 1150 calories

CONCLUSION

As you reach the end of this culinary journey, take a moment to reflect on the transformation you've embarked upon. This book is not just a collection of recipes; it's a roadmap to a healthier, more vibrant you. By embracing the principles of Dr. Nowzaradan, you've taken significant steps towards reclaiming control over your health and well-being.

Every meal you've prepared, every ingredient you've carefully selected, and every bite you've savored has brought you closer to your goals. You've learned that eating well doesn't mean sacrificing flavor or enjoyment. Instead, it's about making mindful choices that nourish your body and delight your senses.

Remember, the journey to health is ongoing. It's not about perfection, but about progress. There will be difficulties and failures, but every one of them is a chance to improve and gain knowledge. Celebrate your victories, no matter how small, and keep moving forward with determination and positivity.

This book is designed to be a lifelong companion in your kitchen. Use it to explore new flavors, experiment with ingredients, and continue building a repertoire of healthy, delicious meals. Share these recipes with loved ones and inspire them to join you on this path to better health.

Above all, believe in yourself. You have the power to create lasting change. Trust in your journey, stay committed to your health, and let the lessons you've learned guide you. Here's to a future filled with vitality, happiness, and countless delicious meals.

Thank you for allowing me to be a part of your journey. Your health is your greatest wealth—cherish it, nourish it, and let it flourish.

Bon appétit and best wishes for a healthy, happy life!

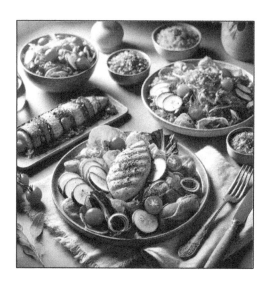

Made in the USA
Las Vegas, NV
24 October 2024

10415269R00050